BREAKING
—THE—
BARRIERS

CHANGING THE WAY WE SUPPORT THE PHYSICAL
AND MENTAL HEALTH OF POLICE OFFICERS

RONALD A. RUFO, EdD

Dear Melissa,

I hope you enjoy the book.

Best always!!

Ron

Advance Praise for *Breaking the Barriers*

"This book is a much-needed reference for police officers. In the United States, there are more than one million individuals involved in law enforcement. There is, however, a lack of understanding on the part of the general public regarding the difficult and stressful pressures that law enforcement officers experience while performing their duties. These stresses have resulted in many problems for the officers, including a high divorce rate, post-traumatic stress disorder, and high suicide rates. This book is designed to provide guidance to the officers on how to maintain a healthy emotional well-being and to help them maintain strong mental health. A much-needed resource."

Cliff Roberson, LLM, PhD, professor emeritus, Washburn University and professor of criminology, California State University, retired

"Dr. Ron Rufo does an amazing job explaining what police officers go through for most of their career. We take incredible raw material, a young recruit who is in top physical and psychological shape, and over the course of a twenty to twenty-five-year career, we basically destroy it. We give these young men and women a life expectancy which is more than twenty years less than their civilian counterparts. We give them an increased risk of heart attack, obesity, diabetes, and hypertension. Along with the physical issues, these young men and women have increased incidences of divorce, substance and alcohol abuse, and likely an increased risk of suicide. That is the compelling reason to read this book. Dr. Rufo provides us many alternatives to help us engage in the wellness initiative, more importantly for police officers not to become one of the sad and heartbreaking statistics, that plague our career."

Jonathon Sheinberg, MD, lieutenant on the Lakeway, Texas, Police Department

"I hope many people read Dr. Ron Rufo's book on police wellness, not only those who are civilians, but also those in law enforcement. I believe if they do, it may save a life!"

Al Lopez, police chaplain, Chicago Police Department

"Dr. Ron Rufo has been a mentor, colleague, and friend for more than twenty years. His commitment to the law enforcement community has inspired me to become a licensed professional counselor and to give back to the community with which we proudly served. This book will inspire and educate individuals on the specific challenges faced by the law enforcement community. Through a comprehensive and straightforward approach, Dr. Rufo has compiled valuable information on mental wellness to serve as a platform for intervention by creating an awareness and understanding of the specific challenges faced by law enforcement officers. I believe this book should be implemented as an essential tool for experienced officers, training recruits, and those considering the law enforcement profession."

Gary E. Kujawa, MS, LPC, NCC

"Dr. Ron Rufo truly cares about his fellow officers, and I hope many citizens as well as officers, take the time to read this wonderful book. Every officer and every supervisor is one of God's most beautiful children, who chose the sacred profession to keep us safe. Police work is holy, and police work is noble. In the last six months, the whole world has changed. We are in a time now where we are forced to change our thinking of planning our lives out one day at a time. We have to ask God for his kindness and to keep us in his loving care. Where our society is headed only the good Lord knows. But one thing is for sure: in times like this, the only thing we can do is be there for each other, not be judgmental, but we need understanding. Not only should we pray for strength after something unfortunate happens, but we also need to pray for understanding. Police wellness is important."

**Rabbi Moshe Wolf, police chaplain for
the Chicago Police Department**

"In this age of celebrated lawlessness and chaos any person, especially one with authority, cannot have too many mental and emotional tools on their belt. Dr Rufo's work here is certainly one of those tools you'll want to place in an area with easy and quick access on that belt."

Chaplain Mike Jones

"Although being a police officer can be a rewarding job, having the ability to make a difference in someone's life every day is an awesome responsibility. Along with that responsibility, the job brings along the baggage of tragedy, sadness, and depression. Dr. Ron Rufo's book is very helpful to first responders by reinforcing the idea that they are not alone. The general public must understand how difficult being a police officer can be and how much we ask of police officers on a daily basis."

Kevin W. Graham, past president of Fraternal Order of Police, Chicago Lodge No. 7

"I would like to thank Dr. Ron Rufo for writing a book that is so important for all officers and their emotional wellness. He does an excellent job explaining the stress officers experience at home, on the job, and of being in trouble even if they are doing the right thing. I am a military veteran and a retired police officer, and PTSD is huge among our police officers; it is one of the biggest factors of mental illness. Everyone in law enforcement should read this book. Everything that Dr. Rufo put in this book is real and enlightening!"

Joe Gentile, retired Chicago Police officer and hostage negotiator

"The mental crisis for police officers today is more prevalent than in any time in history. Dr. Ron Rufo clarifies this in his book, and as something that needs to be addressed and treated so that police are better able to serve the community in which they are called upon to serve. It is everyone's best interest to understand the thought process and the problems associated with policing in our modern city environment. Dr. Rufo justifies some of the police reactions and their attitudes because of the trauma they witness. He explains that there can be a better relationship between the police and the community because, at the end of the day, it is imperative we have that in our civilized community. I believe every law enforcement officer will benefit from this book."

"With tremendous wisdom and compassion, Dr. Rufo invites you into the private world of the law enforcement officer. He speaks to the dichotomy of the 'love of the job' and the harmful incidents that can accumulate over just a few years or an entire career as a police officer that cause distress. He offers practical, real-world skills and practices to support police officer well-being and mental health. If you are a police officer, provide services to police officers, or love a police officer, this book is for you!"

"Officer wellness is a major concern of modern police agencies. Within the police culture, it has been relatively acceptable for officers to ask for or accept help with physical health issues. This has not been the case with psychological health. Asking for psychological help is too often viewed as a personal or professional weakness. For true officer wellness, the erroneous idea that *asking for psychological help* equals *weakness* must be eradicated. Dr. Rufo's book represents a significant step toward achieving this goal."

BREAKING
—THE—
BARRIERS

CHANGING THE WAY WE SUPPORT THE PHYSICAL
AND MENTAL HEALTH OF POLICE OFFICERS

RONALD A. RUFO, EdD

Breaking the Barriers
Changing the Way We Support the Physical and Mental Health of Police Officers

ISBN 13: 978-1-7362021-0-4

AMR Publishers

Credits:
Cover design by Ronald Cruz
Edited by Candace Johnson, Change It Up Editing, Inc.
Interior design by Jera Publishing
Proofread by James Shrieve

To my granddaughter, Alinah, who is talented and bright. Papa is so proud of you. To my beautiful daughters, Rita, Laura, and Cara, who are special to me each in their own way. I love you with all of my heart. To my wonderful wife, Debbie, who is patient, understanding, and supports me in whatever project that I undertake. You are truly the "wind beneath my wings."

This book is dedicated to every police officer, firefighter, paramedic, prison guard, and anyone associated with law enforcement that has chosen a vocation to serve, protect, and help others. To all of my brothers and sisters in law enforcement, thank you for your dedicated service, please stay healthy, God bless you.

The credit belongs to those who are actually in the arena, who strive valiantly; who know the great enthusiasms, the great devotions, and spend themselves in a worthy cause; who at best know the triumph of high achievement; and who, at worst, if they fail, fail while daring greatly, so that their place shall never be with those cold and timid souls who know neither victory nor defeat.

Theodore Roosevelt

CONTENTS

FOREWORD

Ronald Rufo, EdD, has been a friend and colleague for more than twenty years. We first crossed paths when we realized our many common professional interests, which continue to focus on the mental health and suicide prevention of law enforcement personnel. In my role as the chairman of the board for *Badge of Life*, the premier organization that provides education and training to the national law enforcement community, we embraced our common goals.

Ron is a prolific author and is secure in his knowledge and experience as an officer and peer support team leader at the Chicago Police Department, now retired after a full and outstanding career. He then chose to research and seek out the best in our profession to address issues that are salient to everybody in the law enforcement community. His latest book, *Breaking the Barriers: Changing the Way We Support the Physical and Mental Health of Police Officers,* concentrates on the real issues that are faced by our peace officers every day, which include sleep deprivation, family and marital issues, organizational stress, and the devastatingly high incidence of suicide among the ranks. "Being the police" is one of the most stressful careers a person can pursue, and yet these men and women lay their lives on the line for us every day with little open support from the public they protect and serve. Ron represents our unsung heroes.

After I saw Ron's easy and welcoming style, as well as his ability to personally share, educate, and train any size or group of officers, I asked him to train for *Badge of Life,* and I am delighted to see that he continually receives excellent reviews for his work. I recommend that you read this book, which features some of the top researchers and clinicians in our tight-knit society. Please take the time to get to know Dr. Ronald Rufo and the wonderful people who support his work.

To my friend Ron, may all good things come your way and may your book become just as successful as all of your previous books.

With great respect and affection,
Marla Friedman, PsyD, PC, Police Psychologist
July 2020

Acknowledgments

A sincere thank you to the many contributors and experts who have been gracious enough to provide provocative insights, thoughts, and solutions for my book on police wellness. I am truly grateful for your thoughtfulness and contributions.

To Candace Johnson, a well-known and respected editor in the industry. Candace, I appreciate your time and expertise; you are amazing.

To Kim Martin from Jera Publishing for her guidance and direction.

To James Shrieve, a well-known and respected proofreader. Thank you for being on my team.

To Ronald Cruz, a very talented artist who did an excellent job creating my book cover. Thank you for an outstanding job.

To Michael Franzese, a well-known and dedicated author and speaker. Michael is a dear and respected friend.

To Mr. Paul Scarlato for your advice, thoughts, and suggestions which are excellent. Paul, you are very talented and knowledgeable.

To Mr. Steven Decker, an experienced author, for his guidance and thoughtfulness in helping me with this book.

To Cliff Roberson, a dear friend, author, and mentor.

To Phil Cline for his dedication to police wellness.

To Dr. Frank Campbell, PhD, LCSW, CT, founder of Local Outreach to Suicide Survivors (LOSS), for his dedication and thoughtfulness.

INTRODUCTION

Yesterday I was clever, so I wanted to change the world,
Today I am wise, so I am changing myself.
Rumi, thirteenth-century Persian poet and scholar

I BELIEVE A person finds a career path for which they are destined. Case in point, I believe my calling to be a police officer started when I was in my early teens. My dad's friend Phil Onesto was a mail carrier for a short time before becoming a Chicago Police officer. He was rugged and strong but had a gentle way about him. I truly admired him; his demeanor and uniform shouted authority and demanded respect. I remember him saying he made the right choice, and he encouraged me to become a policeman. Living in Chicago all of my life, my first hope was to become a Chicago Police officer. I was recently divorced when a friend of mine told me the Las Vegas Police Department was hiring police officers, I flew to Las Vegas to take the exam. I failed the run portion of the exam, and that inspired me to join a health club, work out, begin a running program, and apply for the next Chicago Police exam.

Failing the Las Vegas Metro Police exam fueled my desire to fulfill my destiny to become a Chicago Police officer. I was thirty-five when I took the exam for the Chicago Police Department. Most law enforcement administration's today have age restrictions on testing and entering the police academy. The trend is to train younger citizens in becoming officers.

1

I felt "déjà vu all over again." The number of people taking the Chicago police exam was unbelievable. It was estimated that 36,000 candidates took the written police exam that year. Out of those 36,000 hopeful candidates only 2,000 individuals would be hired. It didn't take a rocket scientist to figure out that my chances were one in eighteen for advancing to the next phase of the exam. I would have to beat out eighteen other men and women. I was determined. There were three possible scores for the written portion of the test; well-qualified, qualified, or fail. I scored well-qualified. Now the waiting started.

A year or so went by before I was called for the next phase of the exam. I soon realized that any testing related to the police hiring process would be a slow endeavor. I was getting frustrated, and I thought I might never become an officer. After a hiring freeze that lasted a year, I passed the run in eleven minutes and forty-five seconds. My wait was over; I was told to report to the police academy on July 5, 1994.

I was forty years old when I started the Chicago Police Academy. The beginning of my dream; I realized my calling. It was one of the happiest days of my life. I believe I was destined to become an officer, not only to fulfill a dream, but to make a difference to my fellow officers in law enforcement by helping them realize the importance of emotional wellness.

I have been in law enforcement for more than twenty-two years I have seen many good deeds being done, and I have experienced many disturbing situations and horrific crime scenes as well. Many times, I suffered in silence without being able to confide in anyone. I did not want to appear weak or that I could not handle the job. The old saying, "Suck it up kid, you're a cop, that's what we do," resonated with me.

Once I joined peer support and became a team leader, I realized that many of my colleagues were experiencing the same issues that were bothering me. Peer support helped me realize that officers need to know that it is OK to ask for help. I hope one day that everyone in law enforcement will feel comfortable seeking out help and finding peace in their lives.

I am delighted to say there has been a recent increase of awareness regarding police wellness because of the recent passage of the *Law Enforcement Mental Health and Wellness Act (LEMHWA) of 2017, which* President Donald Trump signed into law on January 11, 2018. This act was sponsored by Indiana Senators

Joe Donnelly and Todd Young. This act provides numerous benefits for the law enforcement community by addressing the mental health and well-being of police officers throughout the country. It also provides the opportunity to conduct research regarding an annual health checkup for law enforcement officers. It provides many needed and necessary support-based initiatives for law enforcement officers struggling with mental health concerns. It develops resources to educate mental health providers on various therapies important to a person's mental health outlook. This act will also help identify and review the effectiveness and support of crisis hotlines.

I remember reading a short but powerful and heartwarming narrative called *The Starfish Story* by Loren Eisley. It is about a young boy saving the life of one starfish among the thousands of starfish that were stranded on the beach. I often compare the starfish story to helping my brothers and sisters in law enforcement. Anyone who knows an officer who is having a difficult time emotionally can be that little boy in the story. By getting involved, they too may be able to make a difference in that officer's life when they really need the support and comfort from someone who cares. Just being there and listening may be all it takes to save a life. My goal in writing this book on police wellness, like the starfish story, is to save that one officer who is troubled.

When a person is happy at work, they will most likely do an outstanding job all day, every day. A happier work environment will also mean less stress and anxiety. The advantages of an emotionally healthy police department will not only benefit everyone who works in the department, but will trickle down to everyone in the community. For police officers, this may mean a decrease in overall complaints and lawsuits.

This book is divided into two parts.

Part One emphasizes the previous history of law enforcement and how it developed into our current culture. It also highlights some of the issues that police officers deal with in their career.

Part Two focuses on what police officers and retirees need to do to take care of themselves and how they can promote emotional wellness for themselves as well as others. A police officer who is both mentally and physically healthy is a valuable commodity to every law enforcement agency. My goal is to have every police academy and police administration devote more time to police wellness. I hope police officers, retirees, and their families realize that there are valuable resources available to them. It is important for everyone to put their pride aside and understand that it is OK to seek the emotional help they need; help that will be beneficial to a long and health life.

Hopefully, *Breaking the Barriers* will encourage officers everywhere to take advantage of the many available resources and opportunities that are available to them, many of which are discussed in this book. It is my goal to help my fellow officers lead better and more fulfilling lives, both on the job and in their retirement.

Thank you for taking the time to read my book. I hope this will be a good resource for everyone who reads it.

Dr. Ron Rufo
November, 2020

PART ONE

HOW THE PROBLEM STARTED

–CHAPTER 1–

THE EVOLUTION OF POLICE CULTURE

***We Remember the Officers*[1]**
We remember the officers who changed our lives,
The men and women who protected us day and night,
People who respect for their dedication to the cause,
For when faced with danger, they never even pause.
We remember the officers who always stood true,
Whatever the color of uniform, brown, gray, or blue,
With pride and integrity they say "To serve and protect,"
For the giving of their life, we offer our respect.
We remember the officers who we never really knew,
Persons strong enough to answer the challenge are few,
With heavy hearts we mourn the officers in eternal rest,
There's more to these people than the badge on their chest.
Author Unknown

FOR MANY RECRUITS, walking into the police academy for the first time is making their childhood dreams a reality. The feeling of *I finally made it; I am actually here* is on many of their faces as they stream through the front door. A law enforcement career develops well-rounded recruits with high expectations as they try to make a positive difference in an uncertain world.

---

[1] http://www.mdfallenofficers.org/police-and-st-michael.html

They bring their thoughts, prejudices, aspirations, and beliefs the first day they begin the police academy. In most police academies throughout the United States, the curriculum is top-heavy in tactical training with a strong emphasis on officer safety.

The twenty-five weeks of paramilitary-style training that follows begins to instill in the young recruit the idea to "never trust anyone." This rationale is instilled in every class, every day. The first class of tactical training always emphasizes, "Always watch the person's hands; that is the only part of the body that can do serious harm to you." The chances of being severely hurt or killed are monumental in this profession. Recruits are constantly reminded that their life can be gone in an instant.

The power of always being in control of the situation is the highlight of every tactical training episode. Recruits are told to be that warrior who does not show weakness, and to be leery of everyone because that is the only way to survive! Recruits soon learn they have a great deal of authority and power associated with being an officer. How many officers can handle their authority? Will their newfound control go to their head? With great power comes great responsibility.

Police recruits soon learn they must:

- be warriors
- be focused and in control
- not be the weak link in the chain
- be strong and never show weakness
- never ever show emotion or fear

The changes that soon begin to occur are an alienation of civilian friends, who will most likely be replaced by police friends. It is not unsual for new recruits to start hanging out at bars, sporting events, and fundraisers with their new police comrades. The reasoning is simple: they work together, so why not have fun or "play" together? The new recruits soon begin to abandon what they have learned throughout life and replace that with a new "law enforcement mentality," which means adding speculation, cynicism, and distrust. Some of the downfalls of this attitude include:

- developing an *us* (police) against *them* (citizens) mentality.
- developing an "Are you aware of who I am?" attitude.
- marital problems: officers who enter the police academy happily married may soon experience marital problems due to their career path.
- an attitude of entitlement, such as "I'm special" or "It's all about me."

After graduation from the police academy, the inexperienced recruit will soon begin to develop and embrace a "warrior-like" mentality. This type of mindset could be compared to almost any adult participating in a competitive sport: Win at any cost. Never side with the enemy. Because of this, helping others often becomes secondary because in a short time, they will go from a "helper" to a "hunter." They will soon look for individuals and offenders to arrest. Young officers, if they want to move up the ranks and be noticed by their supervisors, often become aggressive. They try to make more drug and gun arrests. Many supervisors like young, assertive, and uncompromising officers on their team. It doesn't take long for a hard-and-fast officer to be asked to go to a tactical team (plain clothes detail) or special unit or to receive a meritorious promotion.

One thing is for sure: not all recruits will be able to handle the stress of the job as their careers progress. This new approach is completely the opposite of why they made law enforcement their career. Their entire persona will change, and stress accompanied by cynicism will become their constant companion. As a psychologist and former police officer, Jack A. Digliani, PhD, EdD, explains:

> Law enforcement officers work in an occupational world of *assumption of possible threat,* whereas most others work and live in a world of *assumption of safety.* This distinction is one of the fundamental

differences between law enforcement and most other occupations. Officers must assume possible threat in nearly all policing interactions to avoid being harmed or killed due to complacency.

FAMILY DAYS AT THE ACADEMY

I think it is important for all recruits to have their closest family members—including wives, husbands, girlfriends, boyfriends, parents, and children—spend a few days at the police academy. Those family members would learn some of the things that their soon-to-be police officer will be dealing with, and what they can expect when that loved one comes home at the end of their shift. Many family members are unaware of what the future holds now that their loved one has become a police officer. How will they handle what they see on the job? Will they be comfortable telling us how their day went, or will they keep their emotions to themselves? Will their demeanor change? What can family members do to help them cope with the stress of the job? Family days are important to teach communication and let family members know the resources that are out there to help them cope with the frustrations of law enforcement that their loved one will encounter.

Interview with Retired Police Officer Len Cacioppo

Let's face it, when a guy first comes on this job in law enforcement as a rookie, they want to go at 100 miles an hour. As a rookie, they actually develop tunnel vision. They are not looking at the big picture. Many rookies do not notice the small details before them. They try to figure this out as they get older and develop with the job. It doesn't take long for rookies to start to see things from a different perspective; they will begin to see the players, and they begin to notice things. It is growing into this job as a cop. It's like taking baby steps; they need to develop their skills. When they hit the street and they know what is out there, their awareness starts to progress. When young cops start handling different jobs, it begins to test their metal. It is then they realize that they were made to do this job. I knew that I was right for this job as a police officer, knowing that others would most likely be terrified of many situations that occur on the job.

The next three scenarios happened to me. I had been on the job as a police officer for ten months. The scenarios occurred within a week and a half of each other when I was a fairly new police officer working alone.

First Scenario

I was taken from my training officer and put on a car on days by myself. The night before I didn't eat. I didn't sleep; I was a nervous wreck. My first day working by myself started off fine. I started my beat in Uptown in the Foster Avenue District in Chicago, then it started getting busy. I got a call of a man holding a boy hostage at a high-rise building at Sheridan and Lawrence. There were no other cars available. The dispatcher said they would send a sergeant, but back then it was customary to wave the sergeant off; no one would ever bother the supervisor. When I was in the police academy, they told all the recruits that when they got on the street, "You are the chief of police on your beat, so take care of your beat, police it," and that's it. So, I waved the sergeant off. When I went into the building, there was a security guard from the Chicago Housing Authority who said that up on the eighth floor was a man who was drunk. He also said that the drunk man used to be a security guard and that he had a pistol. He explained that the drunk had an argument with his girlfriend and took a young eight-year-old boy with him when he left, until the boy's mother decided to date him again.

When I was getting into the elevator to go to the apartment, a Chicago Police inspector came into the elevator with me. The first thing he said to me as we were going up the elevator was, "Officer, where is your hat?" I told him I'd left it in the squad car. The inspector said, "I am going to have to write you up because you are out of uniform." I told him, "Do what you have to do." I pushed the seventh-floor button, and the inspector said, "I thought we were going to the eighth floor." I told him I wanted to get off at the seventh floor and walk up because the drunk could be standing in the hallway waiting for us to come off the elevator. I was a rookie, but I had enough sense to realize it was not safe to get off on that floor.

We both got off on the seventh floor, and the inspector told me to lead the way as we walked up the stairwell to the eighth floor. I looked under the door as I cautiously opened it. I slowly proceeded down the eighth-floor hallway to the apartment, which was the first door off the stairwell entrance. The apartment door was partially ajar, and I could look in and see the elderly gentleman had a pistol in his hand, with the child sitting at the table.

As I turned to the inspector to tell him that the older guy has a gun, I saw him walking away, going toward the stairwell. The inspector left me by myself. This was my first day working by myself with only ten months on the job. I was thinking, *I am by myself and no one is coming.* No cars were up, it was just a busy, busy afternoon.

I had my pistol in my hand, I was on my hands and knees looking through the crack of the door. I observed the old man ask the kid if he wants some juice. The young child says, "Yes, please." The old man set the gun down on the counter as he got up to get the juice that was about fifteen feet way. At that time, I realized it is now or never. I hit that door like a fullback for the Chicago Bears hitting the line at Soldier Field. I went screaming at this guy, who almost had a heart attack when he opened up the refrigerator and saw me coming full blast at him. The old man turned to get back to that pistol, but I was on him. He went down to the floor, and I had him handcuffed quickly. I put my pistol in the holster, I had his pistol, I had him and the kid.

We all went down the elevator. When we exited the elevator, the security guard said, "Man, you're like Batman, you did this all by yourself. I saw your partner run out the door. Where did he go? He was a coward, man!" The boy's mother signed complaints; the old man went to jail. When the paperwork was done and completed, I wasn't scared, I was concerned for everyone's safety.

I realized that this was the moment when I was tested, this was the moment when I realized that I could do this job and that this was what I signed up to do. My sergeant put me in for an award, and I was never written up by the inspector for my hat.

Second Scenario

I was called to a domestic incident a few days later on my beat at an eighteen-unit courtyard building three stories high. I went to speak to the complainant, who was an older Black gentleman, well dressed, out of character for this neighborhood. He said there is an old white man in the next apartment over who cursed and threatened him every day and said he is going to kill him. The complainant said he never spoke to his neighbor. He said he was a college graduate with a master's degree and an accountant who worked for a law firm downtown. He told me he'd go to work and come home. He said he had nothing do with that old man and he just wanted to be left alone. He said he let the old man's threats roll off his back every day, "But today," he told me, "his threats were with a vengeance. He sounded like he would actually kill me today."

I went to speak to the person making the threats. He was an old white guy, with a Lucky Strike cigarette hanging out of his mouth, wearing a tattered T-shirt and pants. He told me, "Go ahead put the cuffs on me, because I am going to kill that Black guy. I don't like him and I don't care, in fact, I don't like anyone. I'm going to tell you something. I was standing by my balcony doors. I have an Uzi with a thirty-round clip with 45-caliber ammunition, two 357 revolvers, and a 9-millimeter handgun and a lot of ammo. I knew my Black neighbor was going to call the police, and I had the Uzi in my hand. When I saw you coming into the courtyard, I was thinking about executing you right away. I saw you and you just looked like a nice guy, and I decided not to kill you today."

I put the handcuffs on him, confiscated his weapons and ammo, called for another car for an assist. I called the detectives to get the proper charges. This guy was a lunatic. His plan for that day was to kill me, his Black neighbor, and whoever would have been at the wrong place at the wrong time. The hair on the back of my neck stood up after he said that. Sometimes with the grace of God we go. That is the nature of this job. You come to the fork in the road; is this your passion? Is this your life's calling? Or should you find another profession?

Third Scenario

I was working days by myself in the same twenty-eight-day period. Back then we would switch watches every twenty-eight days. We went from midnights to afternoons to days. Again, it was a busy afternoon, cars were all down handling other jobs, even the sergeants were busy. I got a call of a domestic; usually it is a two-man job. At that time, we were working one-man cars. I remember an old-timer on the job said to me, "Kid, always carry two guns with you. If you get into a situation, there would not be enough time to reload." We carried six-shot revolvers at the time. When I started working by myself, I put a six-shot revolver on my ankle, it was summertime and I did not want to have to worry about two guns on my gun belt. As I was going into the building, and I do not know why, but I pulled my small snub-nose revolver out of my holster.

After the incident with the inspector, I carried my hat with me. So, I had the snub-nosed revolver inside of my hat. I went up three flights of stairs, and a middle-aged Black woman opened the door, she had a black eye and her lips were all puffed up, and her nose was bleeding and broken. She said, "I can't take it no more, he just got out of prison, he beats me, he's drunk, I can't take it no more, please take him to jail before he kills me." The apartment had only three rooms, and I went to talk with her husband in the kitchen, who is a six-foot-four-inch tall and large Black male about 220 pounds, who is solid and had a body like it was chiseled out of concrete from working out at Statesville prison. He was in a T-shirt and boxer shorts. He had a big cleaver in his hand, and he was chopping up a chicken in the sink. I asked him to put the cleaver down and turn around. He turns around with the cleaver in his hand and he looks at me and said, "By the time I come over there, I am going to cut you in half before you can reach for your gun, I am going to cut you in half today."

I had my hat in my hand, hiding my snub-nose revolver, and I pulled up the snub and drew the hammer back and said, "If you take one step, I am going to drop you like a bag of dirt." He looked at me, and we locked eyes for a second that felt like an hour. He looked at me, and I could see his gears spinning, *Is he going or is he not going?* I stood there, as steady as possible. I held my ground and he held his ground, and at that time he started laughing. He threw the cleaver in the sink said, 'You got me today, you outslicked me. I respect that, and I will go to jail peacefully.' I made him kneel down, put his hands-on top of his head. I put my gun to the back of his head and I told him, 'If you move, I will kill you, I promise you that.' He said, 'I'm going peacefully.' I had him slowly get up and put on his pants, then I handcuffed him and took him to the station. The guy was a gentleman and never said one word. Even after that incident, I never thought for a minute about leaving this job. If anyone had any second thoughts about being a cop, these would have been the incidents that would have changed their mind.

I had a great career and did my job for over thirty years. I always took pride in my work as a police officer. Back in the day, forty years ago, we donned many hats; you were a minister, a marriage counselor, a psychologist, you did everything. That was the nature of the job. Back then we saved many marriages. We were able to speak with couples who were having problems. They listened and respected the police. At one time, the Chicago Police Department was considered elite, and it was copied for years. Other police departments wanted to police like Chicago, but as time has gone on things have changed.

If an officer back then sought out help or asked for help, the department took their gun and star away from them. The officer was only left with an ID. They also took away the officer's weapons. They couldn't work, at that point they would be lucky to keep the job as a police officer. That would even affect the officer going back to civilian life. The only way a cop sought help was at the end of their shift they would often go for a couple of beers and talk about it with their fellow officers. They would go to the bar and only say what happened to them. The rest of the guys would slap them on the back and say, "Welcome to the club, kid, it is not going to get any better from here on out, this is what you signed up for, this is what your job is." There may be some great things that happen, and then there are days that test your metal, you may have to fight for your life. There were days that I went home after my tour that I went home crying. I looked at what transpired with some of these victims and babies [who] were beat up and tortured that did not have a chance. I have met some great people and made some great friends on this job, and that's what this job really is all about. I am proud of my career in the Chicago Police Department.

HISTORY OF POLICE CULTURE

The culture of policing has changed throughout the years. I mention the earlier years in law enforcement for a few reasons. There were many devoted officers who cared about their badge, but there were many officers who were corrupt and used their position to exploit others. These dishonest officers gave law enforcement a bad name, where everyone in law enforcement were pinned as immoral and malevolent.

1920s and 1930s
When Prohibition was in its heyday in the 1920s and early 1930s, many cops were influenced by criminal activity, money, and greed. There were a number of officers during this time in history who were more likely to use the power of the badge for their own benefit. Instead of protecting the citizens, a good number of police officers who were sworn to serve and protect often turned a

blind eye on crime and corruption, benefiting handsomely from bribes they would receive. This was the era of Prohibition that brought a new meaning to wrongdoing as it fueled Al Capone and other crime figures into organized crime. Graft, greed, and transgression were rampant. Police corruption in the 1920s and 1930s was widespread and chaotic in almost every city and state throughout the country. During this period in history, it was often difficult to differentiate between the police officers and the criminals.

Police officers had the best of both worlds. They had a uniform, a badge, a gun, and authority to take advantage of any situation, legal or not. Even if an officer was caught stealing or taking money, his supervisor most likely was on the take as well or looked the other way. Judges and politicians were also involved in corruption and illegal activity or were even on the payroll of influential mob families and gangsters. A few police officers may have provided muscle for those involved in criminal activity that occurred during Prohibition. This kind of cooperation may have included tipping off gangsters that police were planning an impending raid on a speakeasy or warehouse full of liquor, or just looking the other way and not getting involved when a crime occurred.

1940s and 1950s

The culture of policing has changed throughout the years. Roll call was a place to learn from older officers what was happening in the community. There were many cops walking the beat. They knew who the good people were as well as the petty thieves who were up to no good. They knew everything that was happening on their beat. Rookies often learned policing from their older counterparts, and they would often only speak when spoken to and rarely voiced their opinion about policing.

Graft and greed were still part of the culture, but not as prevalent as they used to be. If an officer was dishonest, it was common for his fellow officers to look the other way and not get involved. Because there were no cameras or recording devices as there are today, it was a citizen's word against the officer's word. It was difficult to prove that an officer was corrupt or doing anything illegal and citizens feared for their life if they came forward. Many citizens would not complain for fear of retaliation by the officer or his companions. There may have been a good possibility that the supervisor taking the complaint may not have pursued any disciplinary action against the officer. Officers were often not held accountable for their actions.

It was not uncommon for a few officers to socialize after work no matter what time their shift ended. Some officers made a hobby visiting their favorite bar after every shift. Many older, retired officers have told me that it was not unusual for a few officers who were at the bar all night to go right into work. A few older officers said there were times when officers would either come to roll call smelling of alcohol and were inebriated, or would drink while on duty. It was not uncommon for a supervisor to take care of the officer who was drinking by taking them home and rarely reprimanding them. Drinking was often the coping mechanism that helped them deal with another day on the job. Alcohol was that "person" they confided in. It did not surprise me to learn that many officers at the time were functioning alcoholics.

Michael Hughes, retired Chicago Police detective, shared the following story:

> I came on the job in 1968 right out of the army after the Vietnam war. The police culture at that time was more of a military environment: listen, be quiet, and do as you are told. Every officer in the district had your back. The camaraderie was probably the strongest at that time. It was actually fun to be on the job. Every month we changed shifts every twenty-eight calendar days. Our shifts went counterclockwise, from midnights to afternoons, afternoons to days, and days to midnights. Every district had watch parties at shift change, where guys would hang out after work, drink, and joke around. This shift change kept the entire team together, and it was fun to be a part of a team. They had each other's backs in every situation. I knew guys who drank a lot after work, and a few guys drank on duty. It was tolerated. They may have sent a guy home. If an officer had alcohol on his breath, we had to alter the way we worked, or had to make sure he wasn't put into the situation with the public.
>
> When I first came on the job, I was surprised to learn a few cops in the district took money on street stops. One thing I remember was another accepted practice of the wagon

men accepting money for bringing dead bodies to the funeral home. That was just the way it was. Some officers assisted area businesses by helping then when they opened and when they closed. They collected a few dollars from the businesses as a thank you. It was just a way of doing business in Chicago, and that occurred in many city agencies, not just the police department. It was the cost of doing business. Some of the guys in the traffic division were like bandits without a mask, and often they would kick up some money upstairs to their superiors. Officers still had to bring in a certain number of tickets. I remember a guy called Cadillac Charlie; he got that nickname because he would only stop Cadillacs and Lincolns because owners of those cars most often had a few dollars. The city wasn't paying much, and it was a way to augment their income, the city knew what was going on.

1960s and 1970s

Police corruption in the 1960s and 1970s was not as obvious as it was in previous years. Camaraderie was more apparent as officers began to bond together in unity with each other. In my opinion, this was the time where that blue code of honor began. All for one and one for all, the officers would begin to fight crime together and began to be one cohesive group.

The police culture of the 1960s and 1970s still painted a grim picture in the eyes of the community, especially when coupled with a few outbursts of police brutality. Officers were known to protect their own no matter the circumstances, even if they had to falsify a report or look the other way if anything came up missing during an investigation. "I didn't see anything and I do not remember." Who would question them? They were the police. An officer's report often vindicated any police involvement. Any sort of verbal abuse or police misconduct was often dismissed and was rarely brought up, mentioned, or pursued. Rarely did anyone question their motives or tactics. Many officers felt that it was an honorable profession, but there were a few officers who crossed the line because they could.

Detectives were also known to help a fellow officer who died of suicide. They might have said that the gun went off when the officer was cleaning their weapon. This would protect the dignity of the officer in a number of ways. The family would still be spared the atrocity of knowing their loved one died because of suicide, and the family would still be able to receive benefits and insurance money. That's just the way things were done; it was made to look like an accident.

Politics has been and will always be prevalent within every police department across the country. Politicians have thrived on the power and influence they have in the police department. They have been known to get a family member or friend a job as a police officer, to have an officer moved to a better unit or district, or have an officer promoted meritoriously.

On April 4th, 1968, the entire country experienced racial tension with the death of Martin Luther King Jr. With the death of Dr. King, chaos followed in many major cities across the United States. In Chicago, many people took to the streets with the intention of destroying everything in sight. Many neighborhoods on the west side of the city and many businesses were ravaged by looting and fire. I was fourteen years old at the time, and I remember the destruction in Chicago as the police officers were diligently trying to keep everyone safe and enforce law and order. It was similar to what is happening in our society again today. Police officers tried in vain to curb all the criminal activity that was occurring on a daily basis. I remember Mayor Richard J. Daley giving the order to all of the Chicago Police Officers under his command: "Shoot to kill."

In 1968, many cities throughout the United States were facing the same political turbulence, civil unrest, rioting, and looting. We are experiencing the same unrest and hatred for the police fifty years later. Following the assassination of Martin Luther King Jr., racial tension, bias, and bigotry became entrenched in many departments across the country. The tension between civilians and law enforcement was never so high. This was a time of great divide across our great nation. We were a nation divided by color, hate, and war. There were daily TV news reports of the clashes between police and protesters on college campuses and on the streets of major cities. It seemed like a weekly occurrence to see neighborhoods and businesses being burned to the ground, looters running with merchandise from trampled storefronts, chaos and civil unrest throughout the nation on almost every TV channel and on every headline on the daily newspapers. The demands on law enforcement were shocking and disturbing, often in a negative way, throughout the nation.

The summer of 1968 was long and hot, as tensions began to flare up once again when the Democratic National Convention was hosted by Chicago from August 26th through the 29th. The entire world experienced a horrifying scene as many young people came to Chicago to protest the Vietnam war, with the true intention of disrupting the convention by protesting and rioting. Politicians were nervous as large crowds gathered and emotions ran high. Warnings were issued that law enforcement would not tolerate any trouble or misconduct. This warning only seemed to infuriate the protesters and demonstrators more. Again, the Chicago Police officers had strict orders to do whatever they needed to do to control the situation.

The television screen was filled with Chicago Police officers using nightsticks, tear gas, and whatever physical force necessary to keep the peace and restore order in the city. It was not unusual to see police officers beating a perpetrator or demonstrator to get their message across that breaking the law would not be tolerated. It was obvious at this time that law enforcement was a force to be reckoned with, and there were little or no repercussions for their actions. It was a terrible time of civil and racial unrest as the cloak of destruction and tension fell upon the city of Chicago once again. The police station lockup and county jail were filled with unruly protesters and offenders who broke the law and defied police orders. The police were praised by some and admonished by others in their quest to maintain order.

In the mid-1970s, many police departments across the nation began to incorporate an Internal Affairs Division (IAD) within their department in order to "police the police." The Internal Affairs Unit was (and is) made up of police officers who document and review allegations of police misconduct. A citizen can make a complaint against any officer at any time. This unit determines if an officer was involved in any criminal behavior, misconduct, planting of drugs, or excessive force and verbal abuse accusations, medical roll abuse, drug or substance abuse, residency allegations, or other infractions of police misconduct.

Many officers invariably did not trust anyone working in this unit. A fair number of officers believe they cannot be friends with officers in this unit because they may be investigated at some point in their career. My philosophy is if an officer has not done anything wrong or questionable in their career, there should be no fear of anyone in the Internal Affairs Division. I really believe that many officers in this unit will do their due diligence and be fair in their investigation to prove the officer was justified in their actions. In my opinion, if the officer was wrong, they must accept the consequences of their actions whatever the outcome.

All officers are given a set of rules and regulations set forth by the Chicago Police Department that they are accountable for. To enforce these rules and regulations, the Office of Professional Standards (OPS) was created in 1974. It is a part of the 13,500 member police department, but it is staffed by civilians. The Chicago Police Department is required to notify OPS when they receive excessive force complaints, domestic disputes that involve police officers, all police-involved shootings, and any citizen-related deaths that occur while in police custody. The OPS unit will ensure that any Chicago Police officer will be severely reprimanded and will recommend suspension or firing of any officer who engage in illegal activity, inappropriate behavior, or conduct unbecoming of an officer.

Being a police officer during this time had its benefits and perks. Citizens enjoyed having the police in their neighborhood, and beat cops were prevalent mostly in the business districts. People felt safe knowing the police were always nearby. Officers would often receive a complimentary meal or a cup of coffee at a restaurant on their beat, or possibly a discount at any store they happened to visit.

Roger Bay had a distinguished career and retired as a street deputy in the Chicago Police Department. Roger explained, "I joined the police force in the 1980s, and like most officers, we did it for two reasons. Mostly the men and women joined the force because of the love of the job, and secondly to get the bad guys off of the streets. [But] society is different and has changed since years past. It is not just the bad guys anymore; it is now the elected officials and the larger population we are faced with. I do not remember a time before when responsible politicians slandered our good work." He shared the following example.

The first time I felt a shift in police culture was when the media's attention changed against the police after the Rodney King incident in California in March of 1991. This was the video camera footage showing the beating and brutality by Los Angeles police officers. The news media constantly kept showing the video over and over. It began to incite and influence people's opinion regarding the police. People were expressing animosity toward the police on routine traffic stops across the country and would ask the officer, "Are you going to beat me like Rodney King?"

The incident that occurred with Trayvon Martin in Sanford, Florida on February 26, 2012, was an incident that began the Black Lives Matter movement. It seemed like it was a small and localized incident that made national news. The public started attaching that incident to many incidents afterward of Black citizens being hurt or killed by police, particularly if the police officer involved in the incident was white. It didn't matter because a racial rift was starting across America, and it was beginning to stir up racial tension and emotions as the media latched onto it.

The media are looking for conflict even where it doesn't exist. If there is a protest, the media feed off its negativity, and at the same time there is an explosion brewing on social media. By now, any small confrontation between Black citizens and white police officers is sensationalized on Facebook, Twitter, and many other media sources that share information and misinformation on what really happened. Today there are more ways to express a person's feelings and emotions as opposed to fact, experience, and knowledge. Now the media responds to what was said on Facebook because it now becomes an exaggerated story.

Elected officials have to respond to this wave of emotion that is being shared by mainstream America as well. The job of the media got tougher, the job of elected officials got tougher, and everything is now pointing back to the police. This negativity makes the police officers' job tougher. One concern of police officers is the possible misconduct that may appear on video because everyone has a cell-phone camera at their disposal. There are some incidents of misconduct or questionable conduct caught on video, but the majority of cell-phone video has actually been helpful.

I never envisioned my police career would turn out the way it did, but my career path ended better than I could have planned. I had many different assignments and units throughout my illustrious career. My career as a police officer was rewarding and terrifying at the same time. The key is to find a balance between operations, administration, and the community, and providing police with the tools they need to communicate effectively. We have many heroes on the job, fighting every day and every night, to work with the community and trying to help people that they do not even know. These officers are putting their lives in danger every day. I found it so rewarding to share in officer's heroism. I loved doing my job.

1980s and 1990s

Young men and women are proud to begin their careers as police officers. They look forward to doing their best and serving the community, proud to take that oath of office. As years pass, it is good to see the practice of graft and immoral behavior almost stop entirely in every police department across the country. The police culture has begun to change with the times, and it has become more transparent than in past decades. Police administrations across the nation began to hold their officers more accountable for their actions. The news media reported any officer involved in corruption or misconduct. An officer accused of doing something wrong or illegal had a good chance of being fired along with losing their salary and pension. It was during the 1980s and 1990s that many police departments began to adopt the community policing model, where the community and police worked together to fight crime and keep their neighborhoods safe. The community policing strategy (CAPS) emphasized communication by changing policy and procedure to reflect the real values and priorities the community needed.

MODERN-DAY POLICE CULTURE

Today's police officers are continually being trained in community policing and in being more proactive with the public in which they vowed to serve and protect. A monthly beat meeting has as many officers who work in that specific area or beat attend the meeting to discuss key issues and problems with the concerned citizens who live on their beat. Experts are often brought in to speak about street safety, burglary, and robbery. These meetings are meant for citizens to work with the police to eliminate crime.

Technology is growing at a faster rate than law enforcement can keep up with. Many older officers have become frustrated because almost all reports and correspondence that were previously done by hand are now done on the computer. Older officers often struggle because they are not as technologically skilled and may have a more difficult time adapting to the new technology they are hard-pressed to learn.

Modern-day police culture has brought about many changes for individuals who want to make law enforcement a career. Many people question what is being done to get the right person to do the job as a police officer. Does testing for the police academy need to be revamped to find a different type of police officer? The career of being a police officer is rigorous, demanding, and stressful. Being in law enforcement is not easy, and only the best of the best are given the honor of wearing the badge.

Vickie Poklop, a police counselor with the Des Plaines (Illinois) Police Department says,

> Police officers make decisions all day long for the people they serve. That's a large part of their job. They make decisions about who gets arrested, who gets a ticket, which way to route traffic, how to write a concise report, how to converse with both the fragile crime victim and the angry offender, among many other scenarios. It takes a skilled human being to be able to juggle multiple needs, multiple people, multiple agencies all at once. The public expects our police officers to do that well, and they do.

The attitude of new recruits has changed in recent decades as well. Lieutenant Adrienne Gardner, Richmond (Virginia) Police Department, explains.

> I came into the police department when I was twenty-four years old, after going to college and graduate school. Working at the training academy and seeing the younger generation coming in, they are not attracted to this job by a pension, and they are not coming to this job thinking that they will be here for thirty years. Many young officers do not think they will be here for the long term. They feel like it is just a job, and they would easily leave tomorrow to do something else. This is their mindset. Many do not see it as a calling, and it is definitely something they do not want to do their entire life, it is a just a job, not a career.

Other officers agree that the attitude toward police culture has changed. Lieutenant Frank Scarpa, Richmond (Virginia) Police Department, says,

> I came into law enforcement a little older, I was thirty-seven years old, and I had a different mindset of what I thought police culture was all about. I was expecting the camaraderie like I have seen on TV shows. Being older, my mentality was a little different, I had a different outlook on how to do police work. With my past experience working at USAirways for twenty years being in a union shop, along with what I learned and was told in the police academy, I soon realized that police culture wasn't what I thought it would be. There was less camaraderie than I had hoped for, a lot of gossip and a lot of grumbling from police officers. It was not as good an environment as I hoped it would be, but I did love police work itself, and I had great partners over the last fifteen years. That's what makes the police work fun, a great partner!
>
> I came in thinking of this job as a great career, a job I always wanted and I felt I was born to do. I came into to this department already seeing the beginnings of social media and technology. I

started to think that I was too old for this new police culture. What I found odd is that there was little talking, little phone calls, but a lot texting going on in our department. The interaction and communication between officers was not person-to-person, it was more conducive to texting, Facebook etc. It seemed like everyone responded to text messages or on Facebook.

For me, it was awkward. I'm a social animal, I enjoy conversation, the back-and-forth banter among officers, but also in the street. It was always my strength. Technology-wise I was an amateur, I had to adapt and learn as far as using it as an investigative tool. So there I was, the old guy learning the young person system of communication. We can now gain information through the internet, social media, Facebook, and Instagram that we did not have before. The dynamics of getting to know a person, the personal things about each other, what they do outside of work, and about their families is not there. We need to bring that support system back as a department. We need alternative methods where officers can share how they are feeling, what is affecting them, and figure out what they need to get through any trauma they have experienced.

Chris Scallon, retired sergeant with the Norfolk (Virginia) Police Department, agrees.

When I first started, old-timers said they could not do the job we are doing today. I retired last year, and when I saw new policies in place, I realized that I could never do the job the way police are doing it today. Now I realize I am the old guy. I think it is the nature of the job. It changes, and we are only police officers for a brief moment, and in that moment, the job changes dramatically. I remember writing a search warrant in narcotics using a typewriter and carbon paper. If I showed carbon paper to a young cop today, they would ask, "What is that for?" I even remember taking Polaroids of crime scenes. Change is inevitable.

It goes in waves, and policing is a combination of things. Good bosses with bad management, bad bosses with good management, and occasionally there will be one person who will shake up the system and turn everything around.

I coauthored an article, "There is No Crying in Police Work," in which we looked at gender and race as factors in how we measure the degree of anxiety and post-traumatic stress disorder (PTSD) we are exposed to.

I was born in London, England, but I am from a Columbian family, and I grew up in a machismo culture. The machismo attitude in that culture is to just suck it up. I was a medic, a fireman, and a US Navy sailor. I went from culture to culture to culture that did not allow anyone to share their feelings.

When everyone is sitting around at the firehouse, no one says, "Hey guys, that last call really bothered me emotionally." His fireman comrades would look at him and think, "What is his problem?" I never had a conversation about a deployment, even though the conditions were horrific, or about how I felt emotionally.

TECHNOLOGY, CELL PHONES, AND POLICE BODY CAMERAS

Television has made people think that crime and murder can be solved in an hour and fingerprints and DNA can be gathered immediately. There is a total misconception about police work.

Technology has become an important part of policing, predominantly with the application of police-worn body cameras. Police officers were able to conduct business and not be as accountable for their actions until body cameras and cell phone video became popular. Body cam video along with citizens using their cell phone cameras has changed the entire look of policing. In the past, what an officer said when they went to court was never questioned, but today it is a completely different story. Police officers are now more accountable for their actions than ever before. Police body cameras are often worn on the officer's chest area of the officer's bulletproof vest. The body camera not only records the conversation officers have with the public, but it videotapes the encounter between a citizen(s) and the officer. These cameras also have the ability to store critical video footage that can be seen at a later time.

With the addition of cell phone cameras, police officers are highlighted on a daily basis trying to do their job the best way they know how. Cell phone video often has not been kind to many police officers. In fact, I think we lost a lot of respect as police officers when they became commonplace. Many cell phone videos have gone viral over the internet. What a travesty, because often these videos often show a small segment of what really happened before or after the video was shot. What may have prompted the action that the officer acted upon is often kept out by the person using their camera phone. An officer's body camera can show whether the officer's actions were either correct or erroneous.

A good example of an incident that was reported and what a video revealed happened took place on January 13, 2020, in San Antonio, Texas. According to ABC-TV affiliate KSAT-12, a home surveillance footage indicated a discrepancy in a report about the shooting of an individual who was wanted on a federal weapons violation. The San Antonio Police Chief William McManus described what happened at the scene in the fatal encounter between the victim and the officers and federal law enforcement agents that day. The chief's account differed from what actually happened.

As the San Antonio public information office explained,

> Chief McManus provided information at the scene as the investigation was just underway. As always, this is preliminary information and subject to change as the investigation unfolds. Surveillance videos are important; however, they don't always provide the full scope of an officer's perception. For example, there is no audio in the video [the television station] obtained so, you cannot hear what the officers are experiencing. In addition, you cannot see what the suspect is doing so you do not know what the officers are perceiving. The SAPD Officer Involved Shooting Team is

conducting an investigation. At the conclusion of the investigation, the result will be forwarded to the Bexar County District Attorney's office for an independent review.[2]

Body Cameras: Asset or Liability?

President Obama approved funding for a nationwide program that would provide body cameras to all police departments and law enforcement agencies within the United States. Many police departments have issued body cameras to their officers for a variety of reasons. The cameras have made officers more accountable and truthful about what really happened during a questionable situation. This information and video footage can be used to support a police officer's account of the situation, and, on the other hand, can be detrimental to their version of what happened. Body cameras have also become a liability for officers, their departments, and the village or city they work for in regard to lawsuits. Many citizens have alleged they have been harmed or victimized by the police or have claimed misconduct or inappropriate behavior. The footage obtained from an officer's body cam has sparked outrage and protests in many cities.

Many times, the footage on the body camera does not reveal everything that happened but sensationalizes only a portion of what really occurred. The body cam video gives a different perspective and dimension of what police officers encounter in doing their job and what they experience on a daily basis.

A good example of this occurred on August 8, 2020, in Cincinnati, Ohio, where Officer James Matthews, a fourteen-year veteran of the Cincinnati Police Department, was on his way to an assignment when he responded to a very bad motorcycle accident. According to ABC affiliate WCPO-9, Matthews, with the help of off-duty Citizen on Patrol Officer Roddy Williams, assisted the victim and potentially saved his life.[3]

---

[2] https://www.ksat.com/news/defenders/2020/01/22/video-of-officer-involved-shooting-appears-to-contradict-san-antonio-police-chiefs-initial-claims/

[3] https://www.wlwt.com/article/video-officer-jumps-into-action-to-help-victim-of-fiery-motorcycle-crash/12012702

Many officers who have worn body cameras don't like wearing them. They feel that body cameras are just another piece of required equipment they must wear as part of their uniform. Officers feel the added equipment can be considered a safety issue. Officers have an added responsibility and can be disciplined if they fail to ensure their body cameras are always on and working properly.

The idea of "Big Brother" always watching, of always being under constant scrutiny, can result in constant stress. The idea of being analyzed for every judgment call made, and being held accountable for any situation they encounter, no matter how important or not, can be frustrating. Chicago Police Officer Tony Barsano, a twenty-seven-year veteran, offered, "I am in favor of body cameras because they can help us verify what we encounter. One thing I do not like is not knowing what is being recorded and what isn't. The cameras we wear record a minute prior to turning them on. What if I am speaking to my wife just before I get a job to handle? It becomes a little uncomfortable knowing someone may listen to our private conversation."

The added stress of being held accountable for verbal abuse or police brutality is magnified with audio and video evidence. Management can use the stored video and audio verification to actually view what happened in any controversial situation. Allegations of falsified reports or misconduct against their officer can be verified or invalidated. Video cameras can also encourage and promote good behavior, not only by police officers, but by the citizens they serve. Video footage can be used as an important training tool for other officers on what to do and what not to do in almost any situation officers encounter.

A drawback to police body cameras is that the public may experience an uneasy and uncomfortable feeling about being filmed and taped by law enforcement officers. Innocent people and/or victims may feel they will be exposed and in jeopardy if their face or image is made public. Victims of rape, sexual assault, or domestic violence feel they may be harmed again by their attackers if the video is released to the public. There are also a few police departments that feel that funds allocated for expensive body cameras could be used for other needed resources.

POLICE SHOOTINGS

Officers are always questioned in police shootings, and are often made to feel like they are the "bad guy" for doing what they were trained to do. No officer wants to shoot anyone if they do not have to. An officer's training shifts into gear when they are put into a situation where they can be seriously hurt or killed. Their judgment call will take a split second. The wrong call could mean their life or their career. It is easy to be a "Monday morning quarterback." Many questions arise after a lethal incident involving an officer. Were proper policies, procedures, and general orders followed? Was shooting the only option? Did the officer try to deescalate the situation before the shooting occurred? Could a taser or any nonlethal force have been used? It is common that in any tense and critical situation, an officer may experience tunnel vision, focusing on one thing and not being cognizant of anyone or anything around them. As they play the scene in slow motion in their minds, many officers who relive a disturbing experience routinely say that "it happened so fast." Many officers have said, "If I had to do it all over, I would have done this instead," most often questioning their actions if a deadly situation occurred or if another course of action could have been taken. All it takes is a split second for a wrong decision to torment that officer for a lifetime.

One of the most dreaded experiences that happens after a police-involved shooting is when the officer must explain what took place in their own words from when they arrived on the scene right up to the time the shooting took place. Everyone that was on the scene and witnessed what happened is also interviewed. The officer is asked to relive the scenario is their own words, often accompanied by a union representative or lawyer. Dashcam video or the officer's own body cam can also paint a better picture of what the officer saw and experienced at that moment. If the officer kills someone, even if the shooting was justified, it can still take a tremendous emotional toll on the officer. Most police departments have issued general orders that reflect the status of a police officer after they are involved in a police shooting. Many departments have that officer on paid administrative leave while the shooting is investigated. Any officer involved in a shooting is only looking for a fair, accurate, and impartial investigation.

There have been many recent lawsuits that have incorporated an officer's dashcam or body cam video to hopefully bolster their client's case against an officer or officers and their department by providing a different outlook or perspective. Oftentimes, the video footage is not as accurate as one would believe. Perception differences between what the officer saw and what actually happened will most likely be brought out in court. This is what had happened in the shooting of Laquan McDonald in 2014.

Communities may feel that police-involved shootings will be tainted because the officer is investigated by someone in their own department. In Chicago, the story of Laquan McDonald is an excellent example of what really occurred and what was perceived. The dashcam video of Laquan McDonald being shot by Chicago Police Officer Jason Van Dyke told a different story from what the officer perceived.

The community was outraged by the shooting, and the media was given the video only after a court order. Van Dyke wrote that he perceived McDonald as a threat, but the dashcam video showed the suspect was actually walking away from the officer. The officer might have been seen as overzealous or overly aggressive, but it is difficult to say what was going through his mind. I am sure that his adrenaline kicked in and took over his emotions and reactions. Van Dyke probably did not realize that he shot his weapon sixteen times. His account of what happened and what actually did happen, along with the collaboration of the other officers on scene, when viewed by the dashcam video caused the community to express their disdain against the Chicago Police Department.

Van Dyke's regrettable decision changed his life and his family's lives forever. Jason Van Dyke was charged with first degree murder, aggravated battery, and official misconduct, and is serving six years and nine months in federal prison. Dan Q. Herbert, Jason Van Dyke's defense attorney, said, "The entire case was more of a political issue. Jason was behind the eight ball in every stage of that case. It was an uphill battle all of the way just to prove his innocence as opposed to requiring the prosecutors to prove his guilt."

RACIAL TENSION

The same racial tension that officers experienced and dealt with in the 1960s seemed to escalate in the summer of 2020. Racial tension simmered to a boil after the media began to report numerous cases of white police officers shooting a few Black civilians who were armed with weapons and a few others who were not armed. Many of these shootings by police were caught on video and went viral over the internet in a very short time, which the media amplified on a daily basis. The news media added fuel to the flame by showing countless videos of police using poor judgment in a few cases that continued to infuriate the residents where the confrontations occurred. Many of the people confronted by police were involved in illegal activity in some capacity when they were approached.

Here is one example of an officer doing his job by subduing an offender, but then using poor discretion, judgment, and unprecedented police tactics. The incident I am referring to happened on May 25, 2020, Memorial Day, in Minneapolis, Minnesota. The officer was Derek Chauvin, the offender was George Floyd. Officer Derek Chauvin could have used a number of different restraints but choose to put his knee on George Floyd's neck for an extended period of time. Officer Chauvin's actions caused George Floyd's death as a result of Floyd being improperly restrained.

Officer Chauvin's callousness caused many people to protest, riot, and loot in many cities throughout the United States and in other countries. There were peaceful protests and destructive protests against the police. Many Black, White, Asian, and Hispanic citizens are calling for change in law enforcement. The cloud of mistrust and apprehension toward law enforcement has never been greater. Though many protesters have peacefully demonstrated, many radical opportunists throughout the country used George Floyd's death for their own advantage, hostility, and destruction.

Every news broadcast throughout the summer of 2020 was filled with reports of riots and looting. As of this writing, tempers are short both in the community and in law enforcement. The police have been shoved, pushed, beaten, shot at, and have had objects thrown at them while trying to maintain law and order. Some people are using the excuse of protesting to cause criminal acts of violence and destruction in their communities.

We live in extremely stressful times. It is difficult to be a police officer today. The police do not trust anyone in the community, and the community does not trust the police. Because of the hostile environment in many of our major cities, police offices across the country are being more cautious in dealing with the community. The situation has caused once proactive and aggressive police officers to be more laid back. Many officers are just answering calls and nothing more. If an officer becomes more aggressive doing their job, they will have a greater chance of being sued or possibly losing their job. A majority of officers do not want to jeopardize their careers and their families. They are being forced to be nonconfrontational when interacting with the public.

In Chicago in 2020, the police department is not only dealing with the COVID-19 pandemic, twelve-hour days, and working weeks without a day off, but they have a mayor who does not support them or stand behind them. Another issue that is frustrating to the officers is an incompetent and weak state's attorney who lets many criminal offenders walk free without being charged. Chicago police officers and the entire department are drained mentally and physically while the city is in chaos.

Because of the volatile situation, more officers are retiring than ever before. According to the August 17, 2020, *Chicago Sun-Times* article, Chicago cops are retiring at an "unheard of" rate. "Michael Lappe, vice president of the Board of Trustees for the Policemen's Annuity and Benefit Fund of Chicago [police pension fund], said 59 officers are retiring in August, with another 51 set for [the] next month. ... double the average number of retirees each month. ... He said a change in health insurance benefits is a factor, while the police union president blames Mayor Lori Lightfoot for not backing police officers."[4] Because of the recent climate of mistrust for law enforcement across our nation, I am almost certain that many individuals who once thought of becoming police officers may reconsider and find another occupation.

---

[4] https://chicago.suntimes.com/politics/2020/8/17/21372795/chicago-police-department-retirements-policemens-annuity-benefit-fund-michael-lappe

The average citizen honestly has no idea what daily life is like for the average police officer. They don't understand the toll this job takes on mental health. Lisa Proctor, chief of police in Kings Mountain, North Carolina, speaks passionately about this disconnect in a LinkedIn interview after one of her officers was shot and wounded while investigating a suspicious person call for service. He was the fourth North Caroline police officer shot in about a ten-day period (two of those officers were fatally wounded).

> No one, I mean no one, knows what it costs to put one of these badges on every morning. Knowing that as soon as you go out that front door you're an instant target. ... I know of no other people who are willing to lay down their lives besides Christ, the military, and police officers. It is a calling; this is not a job to law enforcement. This is a calling because I can grant you that none of us do this job for the pay. There are many of us who could walk [away from the job] today and retire, but we choose to stay. There's something bigger than us that drives us to do what we do every day. It is a cliché to "protect and serve," but until you wear this badge, you will never understand what that means. It is more than that. It is a passion for the people. It is a passion that you are actually willing to lay down your life for someone that you don't even know, just so that they can have peace in their community, so that they can live, and so that their children can grow up and be safe. What I have seen this past [year], that society has turned toward law enforcement and demonized us over the acts of a chosen few, over the thousands and thousands of us that continue to wear the badge and take ridicule for the actions of others that we have no control over, is despicable.[5]

---

[5] Ron Tufano's LinkedIn page, accessed December 30, 2020, https://bit.ly/3n9dSqm.

Some Thoughts about Police Culture

Police culture becomes a way of life for a majority of officers. I believe good advice is to leave the job at the station. Just how many will do that is hard to say. Many officers have a difficult time doing that. Law enforcement becomes our life. Therein lies one of our biggest problems. Do we ever really leave the job behind? Can an officer ever go anywhere, just relax and enjoy and not worry about what might happen?

I have a question that many officers most likely have the answer to already. When an officer walks into a restaurant, where do they normally sit? Many officers sit facing the door and train their families to do the same. They can't relax, thinking they need to always watch who is coming in. Dr. Kevin Gilmanton says, "We over invest in police work. So much so, that we take it home. Does the training we receive ever leave us? Do we train our families unconsciously? There is no need for the officer to bring their job home with them and this practice takes understanding and patience. If a law enforcement officer takes their "controlling street attitude" home with them, it will cause many problems within the family.

When someone asks a police officer to name their number one priority in life, they will most always answer, "family." Everything they do, every exploit, every accomplishment is "for my family." Most families realize the significance of police work but may not realize the toll that it will take on their family member who is in law enforcement. In the academy, they are told to not share anything with anyone, which includes gruesome scenes they have encountered, or the negative occurrences they have experienced on the street. The philosophy behind this reasoning is to protect their loved ones from the outside world and what they experience as officers on a day-to day basis.

– CHAPTER 2 –

STRESS IN LAW ENFORCEMENT

The greatest weapon against stress is our ability
to choose one thought over another.
William James

AMERICA TODAY HAS become a nation of deadlines, rushing, stress, worry, anxiety, tension, and trauma. Society has become fast-paced, with advanced and demanding technology. Gone is the simple life. Deadlines are created, and there is pressure to get the job done faster with fewer personnel at an inexpensive cost. These words are true for many occupations, but they truly paint a picture of what many police officers live through minute by minute, every single day throughout their career.

Stress is often the cause of the anxiety that most police officers experience every day in their career. There is the stress of always being on guard and cautious in their surroundings, not trusting anyone, with shift changes, court appearances, holding down side jobs, and the list goes on and on. Many have witnessed car accidents, stabbings, shootings, and suicides. There is also the possibility of being hurt or killed and not coming home to their families. They learn early on of the hazards they face in their chosen profession. Even though many officers rarely admit it, in the back of their minds they realize that the next call could be their last.

Stress is a frenzied shadow that hangs over every police officer, and it is a silent killer. Many health ailments such as panic attacks, heart attacks, cancer, strokes, high blood pressure, diabetes, fatigue, and other physical ailments are caused or exacerbated by stress. Technology forces everyone to do everything faster, creating additional stress. Police officers are no different than the average citizen in regards to their families and their daily living obligations, but police officers have additional stress. We sleep less, worry more, and do not relax as we should. Stress has taken many lives needlessly. In my opinion, stress is the number one cause of death in this country. It has been for a while, and it probably always will be. A large majority of Americans just do not know how to relax.

Every police officer handles the stressors of the job differently. Stress eats away at an officer's emotional stability and many police officers ride that emotional roller coaster on a daily basis. A tired and discouraged officer may often take their frustrations of the job out on the public they serve. Complaints can range from verbal abuse to excessive force accusations. Every police department has officers who are known to have a "short fuse" when it comes to working with the public. It is not uncommon for sleep-deprived officers who work the midnight shift to receive more citizen complaints. Even their own families may experience verbal abuse and their short tempers at home.

Jack A. Digliani, PhD, EdD, notes that excessive stress can manifest in a myriad of ways.

> Some of the most common include impaired judgment and mental confusion, uncharacteristic indecisiveness, aggression, meaning temper tantrums and having a "short fuse," continually argumentative behavior, increased irritability and anxiety, increased apathy or denial of problems, loss of interest in family, friends, and activities, increased feelings of insecurity with lowered self-esteem, and feelings of inadequacy.

Interview with Retired Chief Mike Kehoe

Chief Mike Kehoe of the Newtown Police Department in Connecticut was the police chief at the time of the terrible and horrific mass shooting of innocent children and staff at Sandy Hook Elementary School on December 14, 2012. He immediately took every on-scene first responder out of service after they were done at Sandy Hook Elementary School. They were mandated to go to counseling immediately through their department's counseling team. Because everyone handles critical and traumatic incidents in their own way, they were allowed to take as much time as they needed before retuning back to work.

As a chief, and certainly as a first responder, I struggled at times, as did the individuals within the agency's wellness program. This was not only limited to my police officers, but to our dispatchers and our civilian staff as well. I felt that I had to have parallel wellness strategies for them all, but I knew if I did not take care of myself, I could not take care of everyone else at the agency. My thoughts initially were to safeguard the community, my primary responsibility, along with the mental wellness of my agency and staff.

The event itself is an overwhelming shock to your system. An officer cannot be prepared for that no matter who they are. Even after seeing many mass shootings occurring in our country, no one is really prepared for such a tragedy. I recognize that a seasoned and experienced veteran law enforcement officer will still be shocked by a mass casualty event, unless they have experienced it before. Even then, I cannot say they would navigate through it successfully without obtaining some type of professional help or self-help.

I initially felt that I was not qualified to make decisions on the mental health and wellness of each individual person in my agency. It was almost like I was going forward blindly. A police officer is trained in a lot of different things. If a person asked me how a burglary or a homicide investigation should be conducted, I could explain the procedures. However, when it came to what step should I be taking for the mental health and wellness of the individuals who were in my agency, it was different in many, many ways to initiate. Of course, I needed to look broadly at their families and their concerns and the steps that I was going to take.

I reached out to many professionals and others that have been through mass casualty events to see what proper steps I needed to take. It was almost like I wanted a blueprint to follow to do that. It was a struggle early on for me. The last thing I wanted to do was to make a decision that would hurt or harm someone. After a while I felt like I had an incremental pathway of what should be done. We had offers from great people who offered to help at our station or at our first-responder meetings. My aim was to give the opportunity to staff to decompress a little, or take time off to be with the family, and not to think about the task that was ahead of them. This was occurring while our responsibility levels rose exponentially. The mass casualty event, as short as it was, was going to be impacting us for a long time.

We incorporated occasional mandatory wellness checks. We needed to develop relationships with our mental health professionals, which was really key. Cops do not like to talk to mental health professionals; I hate to say this, but this is just part of the nature and culture within law enforcement. We had to start developing relationships even if an officer walked in and only spent five minutes with a mental health professional, or if they wanted to spend an hour, that would be fine too. It was their choice. It was done in a quiet, unimposing manner, and everyone had to do it, so no one was being singled out. Nobody was looked upon as being weaker than others. At the time, we were knowingly peeling away the 'onion layers' on the stigma of seeing a mental health professional.

Today, what is really important for this initiative to be widely accepted and adopted unilaterally is to formulate a healing pathway if an officer is having a problem. We know there are a lot of concerns if a police officer comes forward saying they think they are having an issue. The barriers to a successful pathway are the loss of job security through potential unfit-for-duty concerns, and losing their identity as a police officer by removing their authority, their gun, and their badge.

Police are reluctant to seek help, so police agencies have to start to think about how they are going to let officers know in advance of a pathway to heal oneself. They need the blueprint, tailored for the agency and the individual. One consideration that may be adopted for an officer would be to consider taking a week or two off to see a mental health professional and spend time with loved ones. But most importantly, officers have to know what lies ahead for them, and whatever pathway has to be widely accepted and universally adopted based upon the best practices of the police profession and mental health providers.

Stress can be harmful physically, mentally, and emotionally. Any officer seeking counseling or professional help may often be considered weak. Many officers feel that they can handle the pressures of the job. Many may have considered speaking to someone about it but feel that counseling or therapy would be too risky of a chance to take. Someone who starts going to needed therapy is often ostracized for seeking support. Sadly, the officer who really needs to resolve a few issues may no longer be considered a competent partner or backup. There is ill-perceived logic in the question, "Can the officer who is seeing a therapist not crack under pressure when then the situation arises?" Gossip about an officer who is going to counseling may often circulate within the officer's district and sometimes throughout the department as the toxic rumor mill begins.

EXAMPLES OF STRESS THAT
POLICE OFFICERS ENDURE

The following are in addition to the stressors already discussed:

- Politics within the police department around promotions, special units, furloughs, assignments, details, and shifts.
- Home life disruption caused by not being there and missing dinners, family gatherings, parties, graduations, weddings, and special occasions.
- Side jobs. Many officers hold other jobs, often before their shift begins or ends. Many often work through their family vacations. They do not take advantage of the needed time off away from the job, and often get little or no rest, relaxation, or enough free time to unwind.
- Attending school. Many officers go back to school with the hope of being promoted, only to add additional stress to their already hectic schedules.
- Loss of outside friendships. Some officers begin to associate only with police friends, often abandoning other non-police friends.
- Self-medication. Excessive use of alcohol, controlled substances, and other vices.

Sleep deprivation, fatigue, weight gain, and low morale are some of the other stress-related issues that plague some officers. Younger officers become truly unhappy with the job surprisingly early in their career, and with less time on the job are becoming pessimistic and cynical early on.

In comparison to the fire department, they experience more disturbing experiences as well. I am not downgrading a firefighter's job or suggesting it is any less dangerous or emotionally trying than law enforcement, but there is a difference in handling a call. When going to a fire, accident, or disaster, firemen answer the call as a team, take care of the incident as a team, and rely on one another as a squad. They have each other for emotional support in dealing with the situation at hand. Once back at the firehouse, they can decompress, debrief, and talk about the incident. Even if they are called out again immediately, firemen still can discuss what they experienced together.

Police officers, on the other hand, are normally by themselves, and they will often handle one call after another with literally no time to decompress or process what they just experienced. Who can they speak with and debrief about what they encountered when they are expected to handle the next call immediately? Supervisors need to realize the magnitude of how important it may be for an officer in their squad to regroup and decompress after a stressful incident. The stigma that everything is OK and to just "suck it up" needs to end. We need to address the high toll that emotional anguish takes on law enforcement officers.

Doug Monda, founder of Survive First, knows all too well the impact that a career as a first responder can have on mental health.

> Stress in law enforcement has become much more of a prevalent problem in a police officer's career. We have noticed a culture change that has transpired over time regarding the police. It seemed to get worse and decline with the "I hate cops" era when Barack Obama was president.
>
> I think the biggest impact regarding police stress is there is much more on an officer's plate than there has been in the past, from technology to doing more with less. Officers are working harder, bringing the component of home and work together. One big component many people do not look at is the officer taking family stress to work. Their job is stressful enough, it's a bad combination.
>
> The career has changed from more of a protecting and serving to a CYA [cover your ass], not getting in trouble. We are in a lawsuit-happy environment, and everybody has a different attitude in many different parts of the country. Look at Chicago compared to Florida. The environment in Chicago is much more stressful for the officers who work in the city.

Other professionals agree that stress comes from many areas in an officer's life. Luke Fairless, PsyD, a clinical psychologist with the Illinois Department of Corrections, says,

The Illinois Department of Corrections and most law enforcement agencies have noticed that general stress related to the job has gone up across the board, in particular bureaucratic stress. Most officers have indicated that bureaucratic stress is often more detrimental to their health than other stressors of the job. Some bureaucratic issues include: doing additional paperwork for a simple incident, having multiple bosses and getting dissimilar direction from each person, dealing with different political climates within the system and for each administration not knowing or understanding some of the rules and laws within the system, and not knowing how to enact some of the policies they are confronted with.

Eric Ramirez-Thompson, PhD, explains one reason why stress is so difficult to manage.

The thing about stress and trauma is that the brain adapts and becomes less efficient at shifting between exigent and normal circumstances. The brain literally rewires itself, and that process is called neuroplasticity. Neuroplasticity is a reorganization of communication pathways, allowing the brain's nerve cells to compensate for a changing environment caused by injury, disease, and stress. The trauma response describes the brain's ability to activate regions of the brain responsible for survival, e.g., the amygdala found within innermost region of the brain and categorized as part of the old brain, and keeps those activated; that is always on alert, despite the absence of a threat. The inherent ebbs and tides of police work can produce substantial activation of the innermost region of the brain that overtime remains on alert. Although this partially explains those complex systems of brain structures, in this case, experiencing chronic stress, and in some cases extreme trauma. Some police officers definitely do experience this after a while it becomes more difficult for the brain to distinguish the difference between true trauma and everyday life stress.

Des Plaines, Illinois police counselor Vickie Poklop says there are subtle ways for an officer to deal with stress.

> Police officers are constantly stressed because they are always on the go. Officers are not taught to titrate their emotions. Titrating emotions is where the officer turns the dial instead of the dial turning them. For example, an officer can learn to determine their stress level as a number between one and ten. If the number feels too high, they can close their eyes and visualize a dial with numbers on it from one to ten. With their mind's eye, they can see what number their stress level is registering at. Then with their mind's eye, they can turn the dial down on the stress until the number it registers at feels more manageable. It's a simple and useful tool that be used anytime the officer needs it. Officers can turn that dial down to a calmer place so when they go home they can engage with their loved ones, friends, or hobbies. Or they can have quiet, peaceful time all to themselves. Sometimes just enjoying alone time feels like a respite from the craziness in the world.

DEPRESSION

Depression causes a persistent feeling of sadness and a loss of interest. It affects how a person feels, thinks, reflects, reacts, and believes. It is common in first responders with many years on the job. Depression is often considered the number one reason most police officers take their own life. On a positive note, depression is curable with the proper treatment.

Many law enforcement and correctional officers suffer from depression and do not realize it. An abundance of officers deal with emotional issues because of distressing incidents they have encountered throughout their careers. Many police officers suffer in silence by themselves, not wanting to burden their families and friends with their sadness.

Depression may cause other problems for the officer. It can lead to excessive drinking, gambling, marital affairs, and other addictions. Depression can lead to changes in sleep, appetite, energy levels, concentration, daily behavior, or self-esteem. An officer who is depressed may often look for risky circumstances that could place him or her in a dangerous situation.

Police psychologist Dr. Marla Friedman says depression will cause a persistent feeling of unhappiness and can affect how an officer feels, thinks, and behaves. She suggests watching for the following red flags that may indicate depression:

- The officer appears sad or tearful most of the time or appears emotionally flat.
- The officer seems less interested in activities that once were enjoyable.
- The officer has a noticeable weight loss or gain with a corresponding increase or decrease in appetite.
- The officer is often tired, sleeps a lot, or is unable to sleep.
- The officer appears restless.
- The officer is unable to sit still or seems to be sluggish.
- The officer often has little energy.
- The officer feels worthless or has inappropriate and excessive guilt about things.
- The officer finds it difficult to think or concentrate and may find it difficult to make decisions.
- The officer often thinks about their own death (this is different than a fear of dying).

Gary Kujawa, MS, LPC, NCC, a police officer and licensed professional counselor, says,

> Depression is a silent killer in the law enforcement community that preys on their well-being. I have discovered the combination of physical exercise, stress management, and controlled breathing techniques to be a crucial when treating active and retired members who suffer from depression.

Doug Monda, founder of Survive First, agrees, suggesting that depression and anxiety seem to go hand in hand.

Anxiety is in every law enforcement officer's career. Just driving to work they are going to experience some sort of anxiety because they are thinking, "What am I going to do deal with today? What am I going to see today? What is going to happen at work? What are they going to have me do today?" It is the unknown that causes the greatest amount of anxiety. This is the stress officers deal with: "Am I doing a good job? Am I making enough money? Am I going to be shot? Will I be on video today?" Depression is the second half of that tag team.

CRITICAL INCIDENTS

Critical incidents for a police officer are anything they handle that falls outside of what they would normally handle. That includes any horrendous death or accident, disaster, neglect, abuse, or anything that will leave an indelible image with that officer for a lifetime. Survive First's Doug Monda says, "Critical incidents are an everyday thing. I truly believe that most law enforcement officers today deal with some sort of critical incident on a daily basis. Many officers do not have the proper tools or training to cope with critical incidents."

One Officer's Story
I was doing a suicide prevention seminar for a local police department. An evidence technician came up to me after class to discuss an incident that remains a constant reminder of what he has been through on his job. He said that he has seen many atrocious accidents in his career, but he cannot get one horrible incident out of his mind. He cried as he told me the story.

A mother with apparent mental issues strangled and drowned her two young, innocent children in a bathtub, then stabbed them before stabbing herself to death. All three bodies lay in a bathtub of blood. This evidence technician assigned to take photos of the massacre was one of the first officers to arrive on the scene. Since then, he has had bouts of depression; he can't sleep and wakes up with nightmares all the time. He has been seeing a therapist and said that it has been helping him. Police officers experience tragedy and death on a daily basis. Scenes like the one above are hard for anyone to get out of their mind, and they often relive the situations through nightmares.

A police officer will likely witness many critical incidents in their career. Ask any officer if there has been a few incidents that have bothered them throughout their career. I can almost guarantee that any officer can name every traumatic incident they have experienced within seconds of asking the question. Many officers see the worst possible incidents, situations, accidents, suicides, and homicides throughout their career. What an officer experiences on a daily basis is similar to what military personnel experience. Many just keep it all pent up inside, rarely sharing how they really feel with anyone, not even their spouse or significant other.

ADDICTIONS

Any type of addiction, be it alcohol, substance abuse, gambling, or marital affairs, becomes second nature for an officer who may be overwhelmed on the job and looking for an escape. Any type of addiction can develop from that need to escape: alcohol, substance abuse, gambling, shopping, eating, and extramarital affairs are some examples. Officers may see their chosen "escape" as a release from day-to-day stress, but actually, the escape soon becomes a detriment that will cause them more anguish as time goes by. If their addiction is severe enough, it may take them down a road that leads to depression, loneliness, divorce, and loss of their family unit.

Alcohol

I am sure there are many functioning alcoholics in every profession, and I am positive there are a fair number of police officers in this category as well. Many officers hit the bars every time they leave work and before they go home to their families. They often just need "one for the road." Functioning alcoholics hide behind the mask of living an almost normal life, where they drink to hide a deeper inner problem that they may not be able to deal with. Alcohol is their coping mechanism that some officers use as a crutch, even though it is destructive in many ways. Alcohol in their mind eases the pain, but it only enhances other issues they have. These officers are often pretty well inebriated before they go to bed. They get up and go back to work and the same routine happens again the following day. It is not surprising that many functioning alcoholics on the police department are divorced several times and blame everyone else in their miserable lives—including their job in law enforcement—for the consequences of their self-destructive behavior.

John M. Violanti, PhD., an internationally known expert and researcher on police stress, says that alcoholism has always been a problem in police work as long as he can remember, probably going back to the beginning of police work.

> We did studies that looked at relationships between alcohol and stress, and we found strong associations between alcohol, stress, and suicide ideation. Coping in police work is not easy; look at the exposure, the PTSD, the trauma these officers see, the abused kids, the murders, the homicides, the inhumanity of mankind that they see on a daily basis on the job. It certainly taxes their coping ability. Officers lose the ability to cope in a normal way. They lose the ability to relax, to enjoy life and spend time with their family. Instead, they end up turning to an easy coping response that is probably going to be maladaptive. Of course, the easiest thing they can find to cope with is alcohol to ease the pain and deal with the stress, to make things good again. But it doesn't happen that way. Unfortunately, alcohol becomes a physiological habit that is hard to break. They start to depend on it, and soon it takes over their bodily systems; they need it and sooner or later they are drinking heavily every week, then every few days.

Vickie Poklop, the Des Plaines, Illinois Police Department counselor, says addiction is a result of genetics and unhealthy coping skills.

> For some officers, it may be drinking, for some it may be gambling, for others it may be having affairs. Somewhere along the way, these officers were unable to address whatever anxiety was building up inside of them. Addictions start in the same way, and that is that at some point in our lives, we decided that the drinking

or smoking or gambling or sex filled a void that was yearning to be filled. Addiction lives in the brain; that is why addictions are treated medically. Addictions are a medical diagnosis. With the combination of solid medical and therapeutic intervention, people can live addiction-free. All humans have the ability to heal. We just need to find the right constellation of people to accompany us on our healing journeys.

Eric Ramirez-Thompson, PhD, explains that his background on this comes from his work creating alternative treatment methods for people with long-term drug addiction.

Addicts experience all types of life stressors such a financial, physical, relational, and impending criminal prosecution. The premise of exercising wellness is to utilize physical exercises and physical activity of various forms, for example, yoga, as a form of therapy and to initiate cognitive activities that were counter to behaviors that they previously associated with their addiction. Physical activity has the potential to accelerate physiological changes in the brain; that is neuroplasticity, and provides an alternative to risky or dangerous behavior for those who are contenting with significant life change.

Coach Bob Lindsey, a well-respected police officer who is now retired, has first-hand experience.

I went through a horrible period in my life during which I considered myself an alcoholic. I was a police officer for more than thirty-four years. I also went through a period of my life trying to get away from reality, which never happens. I have been through failed marriages; I went through the most violent history in law enforcement in the early 1960s. Alcoholism, drug abuse, and failed marriages are the consequences of getting involved in something that is overwhelming. When an officer is under the influence of alcohol, they are not fit for duty. It is simple as that. Officers need to ask themselves that question: "Regardless, am I fit for duty?"

Alcoholism is a disease. It is like any other disease; it takes hold of a person, and they cannot escape the inability to adjust to it or to deal with the ever-unfolding events it creates. People think alcoholism is where people stay drunk and make fools of themselves. Alcoholism alters a person's thinking where they may often do bizarre and horrible things. There are alcoholics out there who drink to be normal. They drink not to get stoned or drunk, but to be normal. In dealing with alcoholism, which I did, there is a point of realization that I am dependent. Cops do not like to be dependent; they like to be in command of their own selves.

When officers cannot deal with reality or the pressures of the job, the pressure of raising the children, their marriages, and they want an escape mechanism, drinking in the United States is legal. Prescription drugs are legal if prescribed, but what is not legal is to use these things as an escape mechanism and wind-up doing harm. There are resources like Alcoholics Anonymous (AA). My point is when they feel overwhelmed by something, they need to get help and guidance that leads them to a cure. Health is not found in the bottle, in the drugs, or in the escape mechanism like having an affair. My path involved psychotherapy, which I was involved in for a long, long time, and it worked.

When a person talks about people who have walked this path, they are talking about dealing with a sickness. This is sad; officers with this sickness sometimes kill themselves or sometimes put themselves in a position where there is no way out.

– CHAPTER 3 –

THE CAUSTIC EFFECT OF SLEEP DEPRIVATION IN LAW ENFORCEMENT

Your life is a reflection of how you sleep, and how
you sleep is a reflection of your life.
Dr. Rafael Pelayo

Sleep is the golden chain that ties health and our bodies together.
Thomas Dekker

PROPER SLEEP IS necessary and important, and many experts say that it is imperative for proper health. How many police officers actually sleep well? I am confident that most officers do not get the daily recommended eight hours of sleep that they should. In today's fast-paced and high-tech society, many individuals lack the proper amount of sleep needed to function and be alert.

As a police officer, I averaged five or six hours of rest a night. Needless to say, I always felt exhausted, fighting to stay awake because I did not get the proper rest. My wife said that once I retired from the police department, I rarely woke up startled in the middle of the night. One of my good friends on the job, Steve Young, who recently retired, worked the midnight shift most of his career. We often spoke on how tired he was working that shift, going to court, and working side jobs to make ends meet for his family. Steve told me that his twenty-eight-year career on midnights has drained him physically, mentally, and emotionally. Steve said he is looking forward to many restful nights in retirement.

Several experts weighed in on the importance of sleep and how a lack of it affects the human body. Phil Epstein, MD, says,

> The first signs that we find in history and historical accounts of mood disorders reveals that the number one sign of depression is sleep disturbance. We see this with different types of depression; hypersomnia (excessive sleep) or hyposomnia (not getting enough sleep). Proper sleep is necessary for the restorative functions the body needs.

John M. Violanti, PhD, agrees.

> Sleep deprivation adds to poor health and a poor lifestyle. Working shiftwork, going to court, not sleeping during the day because of taking care of family business and whatever needs to get done. There is little or no time for officers to get the proper sleep they need. Our studies have found that cardiovascular health is affected in the long run. Officers do not know how to sleep well. We should teach them sleep hygiene. Again, this comes down to training. Some officers will ask, "How can I get a good night's sleep, even if I can get only six hours?" and "How can I sleep better?"
>
> Six hours is the lowest recommended amount of sleep a person should have. To sleep better incorporate simple things; for example, sleeping in a dark room, possibly using a darkening shade, going to bed at the same time, and getting up at the same time. These things matter if a person is going to increase their quality of sleep. Research shows us that the quality of sleep that police officers receive is terrible. Not only do they not sleep long, they do not sleep well. A lot of this, I think, has to do with time limitations and stress. It is hard for an officer to fall asleep when

they come home after an afternoon shift or a night shift. They walk in the house wound up from their shift, they don't have time with their family, and when they try to go to bed trying to go to sleep becomes more difficult.

Denise M. Coyle LMFT, CTS, agrees that sleep hygiene is absolutely critical.

If there is one thing I try to focus on, first and foremost is getting a good night's sleep. If there is anything the police department can do to allow officers to get a semi decent sleep routine, they need to do it. Many studies that have been done have shown that sleep deprivation can start to lead to higher cortisol levels and an increase in stress levels, agitation, and reactivity. Everything in mental health works and functions so much better if there is a decent night's sleep. Having classes on sleep hygiene will be the first weapon against any kind of mental health issues. This includes PTSD, anxiety, depression, any of it.

Bruce Sokolove, aka Coach Sok, who retired after forty-three years in law enforcement, says,

Sleep deprivation is prevalent today in law enforcement; lousy scheduling, lack of turnaround time, sometimes rotating shifts, court calls, and the next thing that we know we have a bunch of zombie cops out there. If an individual is working more than twenty-four hours, that is the cognitive equivalent of a .08 blood alcohol level. We will not let cops go out on the street under the influence of alcohol, but we do it by default when our policies, our scheduling, and our procedures minimize the potential of cops on short sleep cycles hitting the streets. That's a problem.

When I was a watch commander, I was a huge advocate of what I call the tactical nap, and I will tell the story that illustrates why. I had twenty-eight uniformed officers assigned to my watch.

We worked six at night until four in the morning. We went off duty at 0400, Sunday for the next seventy-two hours. We only worked the four busiest days of the week, with high calls for service including a lot of in-progress runs. The squad was busy. Having said that, let's look at the metric. They got off at 0400 on Sunday, and everyone tried to get family time in—decompression time, maybe including religious services and family dinner. Many had court calls on Monday, Tuesday, and sometime Wednesday. The court could run in the late afternoon on Wednesday, after which my officers would come straight to the station and try to rest there as best they could before their shifts began at 1730 hours. I would find out which officers had little sleep and cut their tour of duty early. A solid leader understands that if they take care of their officers, they can take care of the shift.

The real problem is scheduling power watches that have to be maintained, court calls, administrative meetings, team training, etc. This has a cumulative effect. When dealing with fatigue, many cops are in denial. "I'm fine, I'll be OK," they'll say. No, they are not fine, they are not as cognitively as sharp as they need to be. It is not their fault. It is from the lack of quality rapid eye movement (REM)—deep sleep they do not receive.

Steve James, PhD, a research specialist in sleep deprivation, has some additional insights.

The number one occupation in the United States for the amount of true night shifts that go through that midnight hour is law enforcement. So from a sleep deprivation point of view, police get hit the hardest. Think about it, society is 24-7; we cannot get around not having the police work. It is the nature of the job. What we look at in our lab is how do we protect the officer in the moment from making errors, accidents, latent decisions that could be career-ending or life-ending. We look at how we can protect police officers' long term. Because working at night and working shift work is not good for their physical health or psychological health. We are diurnal (active during the day) animals, which is the opposite of nocturnal (active at night) animals. We are biologically driven to be awake during the day and to sleep at night. Everything we do that is counter to that comes with a cost. The cost is either performance-, safety-, or health-related.

A paper we published two years ago explains the horrible things that happen to the human body when we work at night. We know that policing is 24/7. Officers have to work at night. Graveyard shift officers have this chronic level of fatigue, and even on their days off, they are still not refreshed and are not at 100% because they cannot get enough sleep. They are sleeping at a time of day that their bodies are not designed to sleep.

An individual officer out on the street, their supervisors, and their leadership, need to understand that working people at night has risks associated with it. Every leader, supervisor, or manager should be aware of the risks their officers face. They should support their staff, colleagues, and officers to minimize these risks where possible. My background is in the British Army. I retired after ten years as an infantry soldier and thirteen years as an officer. I have been on the rough end of sleep deprivation, shift work, and rotating shifts. I was never a cop but worked along police officers doing police services. We never thought about sleep. We worked out, we trained, and got our skills training done. If anyone couldn't handle the long hours or the sleep deprivation, we considered them weak. That is not the way to think about things in regards to mental health and post-traumatic stress. We are seeing these now as job-related injuries.

We have to stop seeing sleep deprivation as a weakness. We are human. We have these biological limits hardwired into our DNA. Some people are marginally better, but not immune to [the consequences of sleep deprivation from] handling rotating shifts and working night shifts. Some people are generally morning people, who we call larks. Some are owls, who can push later in the evening hours and still function sufficiently. No one is immune to the effects of sleep deprivation or sleep restrictions. We need to start protecting individual officers' safety and performance in relationship to fatigue.

We need to start a cultural shift with regard to fatigue. Being sleep deprived has some of the same effects to performance as being drunk. Being awake for twenty-four hours effects tasks such as driving to the same extent as blowing a .10 in a breathalyzer for alcohol. If we don't accept officers being drunk on the job, we should not accept officers being sleep deprived on the job either. We want to make sure that they can get home safe. Consider an officer who is on a twelve-hour shift. They wake up, have a shower and breakfast, so that's fourteen hours awake if there aren't any underlying sleep issues. Add overtime to that and that officer is pushing sixteen, seventeen, eighteen hours, and then an hour-long commute home. Now that is getting incredibly dangerous.

Agencies need to consider what they are doing to protect their officers. The impact of cumulative night shifts takes its toll on police officers, and it just gets worse shift after shift. I had the unfortunate honor last year of going to a sheriff's department in New England where a corrections officer deputy logged eighty-eight hours that week. That deputy served his community for twenty-three years and was supporting three generations of his family. The officer was just trying to do right by supporting his family.

That officer fell asleep at the wheel driving home after his shift and hit another vehicle. The accident killed a ten-year-old girl and put nine other people in the intensive care unit at the hospital. That tragic incident wiped out twenty-three years of service for that deputy. He is always going to think about the day he killed that girl; his community is going to think of him as the guy who killed this girl. When someone dedicates their career to the community and is put in the situation where they have to choose between earning extra money to support their family and their own safety, they are put in a delicate situation where they most likely put themselves second.

Fatigue has not been considered when looking at policy, procedures, and shift hours. It is sad. When I speak to organizations, my message is twofold. One is to get the message out, the second is working as a bridge between the union and leadership. There is a lot of shared responsibility here. A union at its core should be concerned about the health and safety of its members. A union that does not worry about the health and welfare of its members is not doing its core function. It should not just be protecting that officer's paycheck or their overtime check. There has to be a balance of doing what is in the best interest of its members. At the same time, the executive leadership should be protecting their human capital. Cops are expensive to recruit with background investigations, training, and getting them up to speed. It is an expensive prospect for any organization to spend that amount of money in recruiting, hiring, and training individuals.

Executives should be putting policies and procedures in place to get a lifetime of service out of these individuals. At the same time, there is a responsibility on the community to ensure police officers are happy going into retirement, where they are physically and mentally sound to go off into the sunset. It is important for them to enjoy their retirement. Working shift work for twenty years will not do that. We know that working the graveyard shift and not sleeping at night increases their risk of; cardiovascular disease, cancers, metabolic disorders, diabetes, depression, and suicidal ideation.

One of my colleagues, Steve Belinky, says there are three things that every species with a brain does on this planet: They reproduce (they mate), they protect themselves from predators, and they feed themselves. As a species, if they don't do those three things, they die. A person can't do any of those three things if they are asleep. If sleeping wasn't important at that evolutionary level, at that core biological level, we wouldn't do it. We actually wouldn't sleep. Most species sleep about one-third of their lives.

Getting into jobs like policing and the military, recruits think, *Everyone else has to sleep, but I am special.* No, they are still human beings. We do things like taking in caffeine, drinking Red Bull or Monster Energy drink and chew tobacco or smoke to get over these slumps when we should be listening to our bodies. Maintaining the alertness edge, by working on a person's sleep, and taking it seriously is important. One of the tactics we use is to really stop thinking as sleep and fatigue as a weakness.

By taking sleep seriously, performance improves all the way around. Sleep is needed to be better on the job, just like fitness, shooting a firearm, or driving, or whatever it might be. We wouldn't want a drunk officer trying to do police work, and we shouldn't accept an officer with a fatigued brain on the street either. When it comes to understanding risk, police are in a risky occupation. Officers should face that encounter in the best shape possible to win the fight that is in front of them. Being well rested and being in the right mindset is absolutely part of that.

But there is another process at play as well, and that is circadian rhythm. A circadian rhythm is an environmental, natural, and internal process that regulates a person's sleep-wake cycle. It repeats roughly every twenty-four hours, and it involves the rise and setting of the sun. We cannot get around that, that is how we are wired as a species. A person's circadian rhythm often starts building about 4:00 am. It is at its first peak around and wanes a bit about 3:00 pm. Many people have the 3:00 pm slump. People in many countries like Italy or Spain take a nap or siesta at this time. Here in the USA, many people have a coffee or Red Bull to get over their slump. But the slump is the body's way of saying "take a break." As hunters, gatherers, and farmers, this slump was designed to get them out of the fields at the heat of the day so they would not die of heat exhaustion. The circadian pressure builds again in the early evening, and that is to allow us to have that second effort in the cooler hours of the evening before we start sleeping again. So when officers come off graveyard shift at six or seven in the morning, they may not be getting to bed until eight or nine in the morning. Their circadian pressure to stay awake is already building, and the bricks in their backpack start to come out. They have been awake a long time. They meet the circadian pressure at a higher point, so there are not enough bricks to outweigh the pressure to wake up. We have all worked graveyard shifts, maybe have been held over for training and we are more tired but we can't sleep as long. That is because we are meeting that circadian pressure at a different point in the day when we are trying to sleep. The pressure to wake up, even though we are still tired and still fatigued, is too great to keep us asleep.

In the long term, working the graveyard shift is not ideal. We need to share this shift and share the pain. We should not have the same cohort of officers working this overnight shift, doing ten, fifteen, twenty years on it. A lot of agencies bid for shift based on seniority, but that isn't ideal. They need to bid for shift based on what they are able to cope with both physically and psychologically as officers. We cannot have officers doing twenty or thirty years on the graveyard shift and riding off into the sunset, because they most likely will die at a younger age. Cops know they are not at their best after fifteen or sixteen hours on the job. There are risks associated with fatigue. Many different occupations have all implemented fatigue management systems, because they recognize that fatigue has been a major part of disasters within their industries past. There is no one-size-fits-all solution to fatigue management. We need police agencies to own this issue internally before they get regulated externally. We need to look at fatigue with a risk-management mindset. Policing takes a lot from the body and mind. Working and not sleeping enough is part of that.

CHAPTER 4

POST-TRAUMATIC STRESS DISORDER

Let our hearts be stretched out in compassion toward others,
for everyone is walking his or her own difficult path.
Dieter F. Uchtdorf

POST-TRAUMATIC STRESS DISORDER (PTSD) is a debilitating mental health condition that is sparked by disturbing, terrifying, and alarming events, which may occur after one traumatic event or from a combination of many devasting events. The effects of trauma can last for a few moments or possibly an entire lifetime. A few examples of trauma that can cause post-traumatic stress are accidents that involve serious injury or death, mutilation, neglect, physical abuse, child abuse, rape, sexual violence, natural disasters, devastation, and destruction. Post-traumatic stress is common among many first responders because they experience numerous traumatic events throughout their career. Everyone is different in how they react emotionally and physically to pain and suffering.

Many officers see horrifying and deadly accidents, dramatic and dangerous situations such as shootings, stabbings, suicides, and other deaths throughout their career. It is not uncommon for officers to keep their emotions all pent up inside, rarely sharing how they really feel with anyone, not even their spouses or significant others. Officers who experience PTSD most often have a difficult time sleeping as they keep these tragic and traumatic incidents in the back of their minds.

Post-traumatic stress is also associated with soldiers who have experienced the many casualties and destruction that are associated with combat and war. Military personnel coming back from their tour of duty experience many symptoms of post-traumatic stress disorder. The difference is that most military careers last an average of three or four years, depending on the branch of service. Most police careers average from twenty to thirty years, and that is a long time to deal with critical incidents.

Many clinicians who have patients with post-traumatic stress disorder indicate that PTSD includes both mental and physical symptoms. A few signs of PTSD are anger and a clear detachment from others. Another common occurrence is flashbacks accompanied by panic and stress. These panic attacks can be triggered by an everyday occurrence such as a loud noise, a car backfiring, someone shooting a gun, or firecrackers. Clinicians also note that officers and military veterans have a difficult time falling asleep or sleeping through the night without nightmares or night sweats. A few signs and symptoms of trauma can also be fear, vulnerability, helplessness, guilt, and depression.

Retired Minnesota Peace Officer Duane Wolfe understands that fear is a natural human emotion, but it is one that most officers try to hide or ignore.

> The first article I wrote for [the website] Police1 was called "The F-Word."
>
> It was about the fears that I—that we all—face as police officers. I wasn't sure what the response would be. But, in the dozens of responses I received publically and privately, cop after cop thanked me for saying what needed to be said.
>
> Others thanked me for letting them know that they were not alone in their fears. The one that stuck with me most was from a former chief petty officer trainer at the Naval Warfare Center. How often do you get complimented by a SEAL instructor?
>
> No matter who we are, we are all human. We try to pretend the carnage and mayhem of this profession doesn't affect us, but it does, and that's ok because we are human. Sometimes life hands us more burdens than we can bear and we need help to carry the load. …

It takes strength to know and admit when you are over your head. It takes courage to stand up, admit you have a problem and ask for help. I think Lieutenant Col. Dave Grossman says it best, "No one takes my life without one hell of a fight, not even me."[6]

Captain Matt May, of the City of Wake Forest (North Carolina) Police Department and a keynote speaker on trauma, explains how multiple traumas may lead to PTSD.

One of the points I drive home in my presentation is the effects of childhood trauma, which affects people well into adulthood. Officers growing up with trauma will oftentimes bring that trauma to the job. These traumas, combined with the traumas of law enforcement, set the stage for many problems. Trauma can lead to trauma. My dad dealt with trauma when he was a child, and then he went to Vietnam and experienced combat. Many years later, he was diagnosed with PTSD from Vietnam. When he arrived home, he began his career as a police officer—a true recipe for disaster.

My father retired in 1998 from a career in law enforcement. I grew up affected by the traumas of a father suffering from PTSD. My dad shot someone on the job, but never shared any of the details of the shooting with our family. He took a test with a therapist to see where his range of trauma was, and his results were off the charts with PTSD. He did not know what he was experiencing until he went for help. My father loves me and is still married to my mother (this year will make fifty-three years), but he was a victim of PTSD and didn't know what to do. I am thankful that my dad got the help he needed. I would not be the man or officer I have grown to be without my dad's influence. He was a victim and loved me despite his traumas, and I love him for that.

---

[6] https://www.police1.com/health-fitness/articles/the-day-i-put-a-gun-to-my-head-PoupY1KacQs28Au3/

The ironic thing is, the things that we suffered as children or in the military can often help make us become excellent law enforcement officers. The ability to dissociate, emotionally withdraw, and seek chaos and violence are attributes that make great law enforcement officers. However, these same attributes that help us on the job often wreak havoc on our personal lives. I meet cops all the time who tell me they lived with an abusive parent or stepparent or an alcoholic parent or stepparent or they were bullied or grew up poor or experienced trauma in the military. They bring the effects of these traumas into the profession.

Officers who have approached me with emotional issues, in my opinion, are not necessarily afraid, but they are guarded. Think about it: we go to the dentist, we go have our physical health checked, we go to the eye doctor for glasses, why not seek emotional health if necessary? Officers do not want to get an emotional, psychological, or mental health fitness checkup for their own well-being. Cops are notorious for being guarded and not trusting anyone. They experience mistrust and cynicism, and are worried if they see a counselor that someone will find out and use that information against them.

Police officers are always dealing with trust issues. It is all about letting their guard down. If an officer goes to counseling and honestly wants to be helped, they must be willing, in that setting, to trust their counselor and let their guard down, be open, honest, and transparent, and let the professional counselor, who is skilled in helping officers deal with trauma, do their job. That is difficult for the average cop to do.

An officer's reasoning may be, "I do not need to go to a counselor because they will find out about me." Officers think they are protecting themselves by keeping their emotional issues in, but they are actually harming themselves. Their thinking is detrimental in the long run, which is why we so often see officers behaving in self-destructive ways. Examples include failed marriages, any type of addiction (i.e., drinking and alcoholism, drugs, or pornography), and illicit relationships. Ultimately, many of these officers commit suicide because they can't live with the pain anymore. Those who resist suicide suffer miserably, and that suffering extends to those who love and care for them the most.

Nick Greco, a board-certified expert in traumatic stress, says,

We may be looking at an officer who has experienced multiple traumas, or cumulative trauma over a number of years on the job. This officer may have not dealt with his issues over the years, thus accumulating stress and memories without any respite. An officer with twenty to thirty years in law enforcement experiences tragedy almost every day that they are on the job, and they may not process the things they have seen, such as motor vehicle accidents, officer-involved shootings, child abductions, stressful situations, etc. How do these stressors impact their lives? Officers may often think to themselves, "Hey, I should get help, but I am scared that it will do more harm than good."

When an officer continues with this buildup of emotional baggage over the years, they may resort to addictive behaviors such as excessive drinking, gambling, affairs, and drugs. Doing things that are not healthy, because of the effect of the cumulative trauma that they have experienced throughout their career, these officers become more prone to risk-taking behaviors, drawing on the adrenaline rush. I have heard from a number of officers that a "highlight reel" plays back in their head with the pain of previous incidents they have experienced. There are certain things they cannot get out of their head, and their bottle of stress fills up.

Many officers retire with baggage from the job, and officers in the first year of retirement find it difficult to adjust, and some cannot take the pain they have endured. Some of the highest numbers of suicide for retired officers come in the first three years of retirement, with year one being the highest.

Many officers cannot rely on their departments to stand behind them if they do reach out for help. It is not helping that our political landscape—our mayors, police chiefs—and society in general are not standing behind our officers. We train our officers to be in good physical condition, we want them to have the best training, but we do not think about their mental health and their mental well-being. We put them on the street, with this cumulative stress; how is that not a liability? If an officer has a squad car with a bad piston or something faulty, they get it fixed. So how is an officer who needs help not a liability? The entire argument is that if we do not talk about police suicide, it's going to go away. In the United States, we had 228 police suicides in 2019 alone, and that was what was documented. A more concerning question is how many officers have killed themselves that we don't know about? We are finding a significant increase in suicide among police officers between forty-five and fifty-four years old.

Getting rid of an officer with PTSD is a mistake. They can be treated. The big word here is that recovery is possible. If an officer gets sick, either physically or psychologically, the idea is that they can still come back to work. It is important for officers to get help early. If a diabetic does not watch their insulin and glucose, their problems escalate; cardiac issues, poor circulation, vison problems, and kidney concerns are the result. It is not much different when trauma and hypertension are untreated—things are going to get worse. But there are numerous recovery stories, there are officers who have beaten alcoholism and other traumas, and they are back on the job at full capacity, thriving. PTSD is not a career-ending situation.

Doug Monda, founder of Survive First, says,

The thing we need to be clear about is the definition of post-traumatic stress. Everyone uses this term now like they use the term "the common flu," as in "I have the flu; I have post-traumatic stress." There is a difference between post-traumatic stress, post-traumatic stress injury, and post-traumatic stress disorder. I had night terrors, anxiety, and the inability to go out into certain public groups, all the way up to tremors and the way I reacted to certain smells and sounds.

Every law enforcement officer is going to experience post-traumatic stress in their career, and that stress continues to accumulate over time. Could we handle one incident of post-traumatic stress? Sure, but when a cop is taking on dozens and dozens of traumatic incidents through the week, then that stress becomes critical.

In my presentations, I use a metaphor of a cop pushing a wheelbarrow to work every day. That work wheelbarrow gets filled with every bad incident they deal with. That work wheelbarrow, sooner or later, gets so full that if they move a little bit too far left or right, it is going to get dumped out. When an officer "dumps" in law enforcement, they dump both mentally and physically, and sooner or later they crash.

For example, one of the things that impacted me was my experience in Louisiana during Hurricane Katrina in 2005. What I saw there was the lack of humanity in the way people were treating each other. There was robbing, stealing, and shooting. The number of dead bodies and the destruction was so massive that it left an image in my head. It overloaded my wheelbarrow. It was something I could not get rid of on my own. Cops are not trained to go out and help their fellow officer get rid of stress and trauma. That is not our thing. We are trained to serve and protect. We need to train differently, and police agencies need to hire professionals who will help us clear out that wheelbarrow.

There is a difference between the military and the law enforcement career. I come from a huge military family. I will never take anything away from someone in the military. I want to make that clear, my entire family has been in the military. What I want to explain to people is that when a person enters the military it is a little different when a person enters law enforcement. They are basically both structured the same; law enforcement is paramilitary; there are standard rules and regulations. When a person enters the military, they usually are sent to another country, and if they do go to combat, they may fight a war for a couple of years, [often a] war we have no business engaging in, and then these soldiers come home. When they come home, they are pretty much treated well with many opportunities such as medical and clinical treatments. As a military person, they get a holiday, and a discount at most stores they frequent. Not a big deal, but well deserved.

A cop goes to war every day, a different kind of war than a soldier does. They may not be in a field with 300 guys shooting across the other side of each other. They go to war every day of their life in their own country fighting bad guys—they are in gun fights, knife fights, and in verbal combat. A cop may walk up to a car to help somebody, and someone jumps out of the car and starts shooting at them. The difference between the military and the law enforcement career is that a cop fights a war for twenty-plus years. But police officers do not have the same resources that a military veteran has. They may get a free cup of coffee at the 7-11, but that's it.

Most combat veterans who come into law enforcement have a meltdown much, much sooner than the average cop. They are already entering the game with an injury. They experience a huge impact in their military service; I saw it with every one of the guys who I was with overseas who became police officers. They had a different attitude, they were already pre-scarred, and they did not have the proper training and debriefing coming into their law enforcement careers.

Chris Scallon, retired sergeant with the Norfolk Police Department, understands what Monda means.

From day one of joining the police department, I walked through the door carrying a heavy bag of drama and trauma. After a decade of both investigative and undercover work, I recognized the adverse effects of the cumulative exposure to critical incidents. First responders all exist on a spectrum of exposure, from high functioning to low functioning. The spectrum includes officers who just need to talk, and then there are officers who need immediate medical psychiatric intervention. I don't care if it is PTSD, I don't care if it is anxiety, depression, or suicidal ideation—they are all happening now in any given police agency, in various stages. The only way to start making a dent in helping officers out is to address the underlying causation and the issues as they exist on the spectrum.

After the last shooting I was involved in, I was experiencing depression, PTSD, anxiety, and suicidal ideation. At one point, I got sick and tired of being "sick and tired." There was nothing for me. I was involved in seven shootings over my career, and I was only required to see a psychologist for the last one because I killed somebody. Killing someone doesn't happen a lot. Although how many officers pull their weapon with the intention of killing someone? That happens a lot in a police officer's career. Physiologically and psychologically, there is no difference between the two. For some reason, there wasn't help for these incidents. Once I addressed my own issues, I quickly realized that I needed to establish a formal response to officers experiencing any form of crisis, so, I set forth to create a Critical Incident Stress Management/Peer Support Unit. Every police agency in America is undermanned, so asking for resources is difficult. At that time, eleven Norfolk Police officers had completed suicide in the previous twenty years. Bottom line, we are not protecting nor providing culturally competent resources for our officers.

Sergeant Tom Grutizius's Story of His Bout with Post-Traumatic Stress

Tom has worked in law enforcement for more than twenty-five years, and has been a sergeant for fifteen plus years. Tom has responded to multiple death investigation calls, experienced suicides, homicides, death from natural causes, a fatal car crash, and multiple drug overdose deaths. In some of these cases, Tom either knew the deceased or their family members. Like most police officers, Tom went from one call to the next just doing his job.

As mentioned earlier, one of the worst crime scenes Tom responded to was at a house where a mentally disturbed mother had savagely killed her two twin girls and then killed herself in a bathtub. The bathtub overflowed with blood. When Tom went home that day, he was physically and emotionally drained. A week or so after that horrific experience, Tom began experiencing tightness in his chest, and he wasn't sleeping well. He would get angry at the littlest things at work and at home. He started having flashbacks of the crime scene. Tom avoided patrolling the neighborhood where the tragic murder-suicide happened. He confided in his wife that his symptoms were not going away. Tom's wife suggested that he call the therapist he had seen over the years. He listened to his wife's advice and made the call.

During the first few months of therapy, Tom's symptoms continued. He became hypervigilant and continued to avoid going by the house where the crime occurred. His anxiety was triggered by newspaper articles about this tragic crime. Songs on the radio would bring on sadness and visions of the tragic scenes that he desperately wanted to forget. Tom realized that he had taken this case hard because he is a twin. He received Eye Movement Desensitization and Reprocessing (EDMR) treatments from the department's social worker, which helped to block out the crime scene images.

Tom knew he had to speak with a professional. He initially worried about how he would be perceived by his peers, how long his symptoms were going to last, and if he would project his trauma onto his family and his fellow officers, whom he confided in. Tom struggled with the fact that he might be forced to leave police work before his planned retirement date. He lost his faith in society and in God.

Tom learned in therapy that he was used to absorbing the pain and grief of others. He experienced survivor's guilt. While in therapy, Tom went on many death investigation calls, including two hanging deaths in one weekend, and two infant deaths within a nine-day period. The "death train" just did not stop. It made his recovery process more challenging.

Tom realized through therapy and counseling that everyone needs to be compassionate to themselves and that the most important person in therapy is "me." He learned how to mediate and discuss what was bothering him with his therapist.

"Making a call to a therapist is not a sign of weakness but a sign of courage and strength," Tom says today. He read books on resilience and post-traumatic growth. "My therapist told me to start journaling, and I started yoga," he shares. "Therapy helped me gain humanity and compassion back. It gave me the ability to grieve and be myself again. My goal is to tell other officers that it is imperative to seek help if they are hurting emotionally."

– CHAPTER 5 –

POLICE MARRIAGE AND THE

LIKELIHOOD OF DIVORCE

I grasped the meaning of the greatest secret that human
poetry and human thought and belief have to impart. The
salvation of man is through love and in love.
Viktor Frankel

MY FIRST WEEK in the Academy, I remember my homeroom instructor asking, "How many recruits in this room are married?" Probably thirty of the forty recruits raised their hands. The instructor said vehemently, "Eighty percent of married officers starting their career in law enforcement will most likely be divorced before their careers end, and that number may be even higher, most likely because of this job."

I have to admit I was pretty amazed by his statement. I wondered to myself why there was such a high divorce rate in law enforcement and why nothing was being done about it. Was there that much stress on this job that would cause this much heartache? What was it about this job that changed a person? Surprisingly, no one asked the instructor why police officers had such a high divorce rate. After speaking to many officers throughout my career, I found out that many police officers often refuse to share their worries and fears with anyone, keeping their troubled thoughts behind the locked facade in their minds.

"Every cop I know is divorced. It's a pandemic!" That statement is from Jonathon Sheinberg, MD, lieutenant of the Lakeway, Texas, police department. He seems to agree with my instructor at the Academy that life as a police officer isn't easy on marriages. Other professionals agree and offer a variety of reasons why.

LACK OF TIME WITH FAMILY

Kurt Gawrisch, a certified Critical Incident Team instructor, says,

> If a person asks an officer what is most important to them, a common reply is "family." Yet we (officers) spend most of our time on the job either on the street, at court, or working secondary employment. While officers are away financially supporting the family, that family maybe crumbling emotionally at the same time. I was once told by an officer's spouse, "All I want is time with him." How often do officers forget that families want them around? Some departments have created family days in the Academy showing the new recruits what officers will likely go through in their career. It is important for the officer's family to have a basic introduction to law enforcement culture regarding unique job stressors the officer will experience, such as working holidays and rotating shifts. The family members and new recruits will be told about the available resources and support services that are available.

TAKING THE JOB HOME

Vickie Poklop, Police Counselor with the Des Plaines, Illinois, Police Department says,

> When an officer is good at managing crisis after crisis out on the street, it may be difficult for him to transition from adrenaline

rush back to calm mode when they get home at the end of their shift. It doesn't mean that they are not happy to be home; it just means that they may need some time to settle into their home role. In other words, they have to learn to take off their police hat and put on their off-duty hat. It is wise to allow for some transition time in order to allow this to happen.

Some police officers tell me that the drive home is their decompression time. This is true if the commute home is longer than thirty minutes. This is the time to make an effort to transition from the police brain to the home brain. What does an officer want to do when they get home? Are there tasks to accomplish? A game or dance recital to go to? Who they would like to chat with? Planning the rest of their day on their drive home can help to ease the adjustment of settling back into other roles that do not include being a police officer. Officers are a multidimensional group with varied interests. They get to chart their own course.

NEED FOR CONTROL

Chaplain Kim Davis of the Chicago Police Department says,

I believe the divorce rate among police officers is slightly higher than other professions for two reasons. The first centers around control. We are taught as police officers to always be in control. When we are called to a situation, we bring the solution. When we are at home, giving up control can be problematic in a marriage.

There are some things we can control and some things we can't. My husband, Mark, who's also a police officer, and I have been married for sixteen years. If something happens, who makes the final decision? Working with your partner is the same in marriage as it is on the street. Partners are good at different things. If both realize what they are both good at, they can work in tandem with one another and accomplish marital goals.

The second reason I think the divorce rate is higher is due to the amount of time that we spend away from home. There are times when an officer works ten- or twelve-hour shifts. Long hours can be difficult on the officer and on the household.

COMMUNICATION STRUGGLES

Poklop acknowledges that police officers do not like to talk about their bad experiences with their friends or spouses, so having transition time is even more important.

> If they have dealt with something tragic or sad that day, like the death of a young person or a bad motor vehicle crash with multiple injuries and/or fatalities, they may not even consider sharing this information with their life partner. They end up storing their emotions inside, not understanding that this creates a huge divide between them and their loved ones. They do this out of self-protection and for the protection of their families. They do not see the point of sharing gruesome details that they think will only serve to upset their spouses or life partners. But what they may not be considering is that their spouses or life partners may be able to handle the details. Or quite possibly, the officer may be offered comfort and understanding and compassion when sharing their stories. We all have a tendency to look at things through our own perception, which quite naturally is void of the vast swath of perception that is actually available to us.
>
> When male officers decide to seek help, it is often because they have reached a crisis point. Sometimes the crisis is that their marriage is at a breaking point. When people get married, they do so because they love each other and they want to be together a long time. I don't think anyone enters into marriage and says, "Gee, I think I am going to be here for a year or two and then I am going to leave." I believe people enter into marriage with

good faith and with good intention, but when stress comes, the couple may start to develop little cracks in their marriage. If those little cracks are not addressed, then they become huge divides, which then become huge craters, and they get to a point where reconciliation does not seem like an option at all. But perhaps if things had been addressed when the cracks were just beginning, then maybe the cracks would not cause the destruction of their relationship.

Captain Matt May, of the City of Wake Forest (North Carolina) Police Department, agrees that the combination of job stressors and less-than-optimal communication can cause many police marriages to end up in divorce.

I think that all the attributes and tactics that officers learn in their police training unfortunately helps them disassociate and emotionally withdraw from their significant other. Officers often experience chaos and trauma in their career, and they frequently maintain a level of hypervigilance to keep them alive. Many officers take the traumas and stresses of the job home with them and make it a part of their personal lives. I believe that all the things that keep us alive as police officers have a dramatic effect in our personal lives and in our relationships. Most officers find it difficult, if not impossible, to turn off their officer safety tactics and self-protective mechanisms when they get home. Officers whose significant other has had a bad day may feel that it's nothing compared to the day that they had.

The traumas of law enforcement definitely take their toll on a marriage. It is not uncommon for an officer's significant other to get tired of dealing with the problems associated with the law enforcement profession. It is at this point that the officer needs the love, care, compassion, and support the most. Unfortunately, their significant other has been traumatized and damaged by the hurting officer, so intervention and counseling may be necessary for not only the officer but also their significant other and any children who are also affected. One traumatized officer can affect many people.

Chris Scallon, retired sergeant with the Norfolk Police Department, says,

I been married three times because I am good at it. Home life affects work, and work affects home life and the marriage. I teach a class on how to destroy a marriage; it lasts four seconds and is titled, "Don't talk to each other, just don't talk to each other." I guarantee your problems plus half of your stuff will go away when you don't talk to each other. I ask this of my fellow colleagues during speaking engagements: "Do you tell your wives or significant other the bad things that affect your work as an officer?" Almost 80% will say no. I then ask, "Why?"

Officers often say, "I don't want to put that kind of trauma or weight on my family. I am trying to protect them." I follow up by asking, "So, what happens if you come home and your significant other has just been pistol-whipped and robbed? What is the first question that you are going to ask? 'What happened?' What if they said they did not want to put that trauma on you? To hell with that!" What an officer needs to determine is what their wife or significant other needs to hear. Police are going to see horrific things; that is just the nature of the beast. Do my loved ones want to hear the Disney version of how my day went or the Quintin Tarantino version of how my day went? Spouses need to find out early on about what our job entails.

Officers are going to experience bad stuff, so why not figure out how to address it beforehand? Sometimes when I come through the door, I may tell my wife to give me a second. She already knows that I am processing some stuff; if I didn't have that communication, she might think I am simply ignoring her. The important thing is to tell her that I would rather not discuss a bad situation that occurred with me that day. Having that conversation beforehand prevents a fight later. The marriage thing is simple: just talk to each other and have those difficult conversations at a later time. It is as simple as communication. Communicate what is going on, and when it is a good time to talk. Just be upfront and honest.

Denise M. Coyle, LMFT, CTS, says,

The reason there are so many divorces in law enforcement is because of the lack of communication. Officers do not know how to communicate with their spouses. If the officer has a bad day, they come home, they are in a bad mood, they may pick a fight with their partner or just not talk to their partner. These officers feel as though they either have to tell their partner all about their day or not share at all.

The law enforcement member often will not share a big part of their life or their job with their partner at home. It often makes the couple feel like they are not together. It is not unusual for an officer having a bad day to be cranky and not wanting to talk. Their spouse may keep asking, "What's wrong? What's wrong?" This could lead into an argument. The officer angrily yells, "I do not want to talk about it." His wife says, "You never want to talk about it." He says, "I don't feel like it!!" She says, "You never let me into your world!" This behavior often creates a rift.

From what I have seen, police officers often resort to an all-or-nothing way of thinking. What I have found with my law enforcement and fire department couples in counseling is that they need to come to an understanding. One of ideas I have heard is to say, "I prefer not to mention what I handled today, but I will tell you if I had a good day or a bad day, and maybe a little of what it entailed. Such as I had a real bad day and it involved children, I had a real bad day, and it involved death." Your spouse now knows that it not appropriate to have an extended conversation at that time.

It is key for every law enforcement to learn to create rules around their communication. To create these rules, they need to look at how they communicate, not what they communicate. If this happens, then this couple will increase the chances and the likelihood of having a successful marriage. Explore a healthy *how* to communicate and then the *what* they communicate becomes easier to work through.

Police psychologist Dr. Marla Friedman says,

Officers don't want to bring the job home, I get that, but there is a way to communicate what is happening on the job without contaminating the home front. When your spouse asks about your day, try to confide in them and tell them it was not a good day, and speaking later might be better. If an officer is gutsy, they may also say, "I don't care about the stigma about maintaining good mental health, I'm going to see a professional mental health professional who works with first responders so both of us and our family will be emotionally healthy." Maybe I'm fantasizing about the police of the future, but this really works! Isolation, refusing to communicate, infidelity, drinking, and using drugs is the road to the loss of family. The life of a peace officer is fraught with stress, trauma, bullying, politics, and frustration in addition to the good parts of the job. Make a choice, be smart and proactive, and don't follow the crowd. Getting family help is important, and know that we are here.

Lieutenant Frank Scarpa, Richmond (Virginia) Police Department, surmises,

One of the biggest issues for police officers is that we just can't go home and dump our "stuff," the trauma we experience, on our family members. They don't know how to process it or even what to say. Then those same officers go to work and try to talk to their partners about what they are feeling. They are going through the same stuff, and they do not want to hear it either.

Most of the time we are keeping our problems all bottled up, so we have to create an environment where we can talk to a trained professional or counselor who knows how to handle issues that we face every day as officers. This philosophy will help future officers and police departments change dramatically over the next twenty years. It will take a while. Police officers are macho, they want to run and gun, and make arrests, and have that thick skin. I don't care how thick-skinned they are, it will get to them. It happens. It happened to me, and it happened to my partner.

I have been married twenty-seven years, but it is important to have other activities outside of the police department. That includes friends and hobbies. I do not dump what I do at my job on my wife. It creates anxiety for her. I try to keep my world separate, but will talk with some of my older friends, some of whom are in law enforcement. We talk about the old days, what the kids are doing, and we leave our careers on the side and just talk about what's going on in the world. As officers, we all need to detach from our police life and enjoy the rest of what life has to offer, and that balance will make us all better officers.

EXTRAMARITAL AFFAIRS

Doug Monda, founder of Survive First, offers this explanation for why police officers turn to extramarital affairs.

An excellent clinician named Dr. Denise Coyle explained to me that there is so much stuff in the brain of a cop. When the brain cannot handle it, it starts to misfire and change behaviors. That is usually through alcoholism, drugs, and infidelity. The brain craves stimulation, and these officers are not getting the stimulation they need when they go home. They come home to a wife bitching in their ear about the kids, bills, etc. Most cops have these affairs because they crave positive stimulation. They do not want to come home and listen to the wife bitch, so they find someone who will tell them positive things like, "You're so nice, you're so great."

Lieutenant Adrienne Gardner, Richmond (Virginia) Police Department, agrees.

Officers often seek an unhealthy release, always seeking that constant high, whether it is at work or somewhere else. It leads officers to numerous extramarital affairs. It is an unhealthy way to deal with issues; their thoughts are that they are going to find someone else to keep their mind excited, fresh, and new. They do not want to deal with the problems they face at home. Many officers work a lot of overtime, but I don't think it is just for the money, I think they just do not want to deal with the problems they encounter at home. It is important to have outside activities and just disconnect from police work when a person is in law enforcement.

It is important to be aware of the negative biproducts of the job. Keeping lines of communication open is one way of putting protective factors in place to ward off divorce. Dating each other and keeping the marriage fresh is equally helpful.

Rabbi Moshe Wolf, police chaplain for the Chicago Police Department, says,

As far as police marriages are concerned, let's concentrate on two beautiful human beings married to each other. The only thing a couple in a police marriage occasionally does is lose focus. It is OK to come home and let your spouse know that you are depressed and that something is bothering you. Let's not forget the human element in marriage.

I have three rules in life. Rule number 1: Not every remark merits a response. Why do we go through life thinking we have to respond and make an issue of whatever was said? Rule number 2: You never have to regret what you don't say. Think about that and let it sink in. If you do not say anything you will have nothing to regret. Rule number 3: We need to accept the fact that we will not be able to understand everything in life. Life is not fair, but that does not mean that we should not enjoy life.

Let me share a story: Every October, Chicago holds a marathon. Last year, Jimmy, who is a police officer, asked me if he should he run the marathon. I asked him why he wanted to run the marathon. He said, "I could drink all of the beer I want after the race is over, LOL." Then I asked Jimmy why he did not want to run the marathon, and he said, "Look at me. I am sixty-three years old, and I never ran a marathon before." I said, "Jimmy, go for it, and do the best that you can."

He called me a few days after the race and said, "Rabbi, thank you for telling me to run the marathon, and I learned a few valuable lessons. I compared the marathon I just ran to the marathon of life. I realize that not all of us are going to make it to the finish line. I realized that not all of us are equipped to make it to the finish line. I realized that some of us are better equipped to run than others." He then started crying, and he said, "Moshe, this is what happened. As I was running, I noticed a guy without feet in the wheelchair watching the runners go by. Each time I wanted to quit, I thought about that guy in the wheelchair. I thought he would do anything to have a pair of feet and be able to run the marathon. I realized how blessed I am. All the way to the finish line, I noticed many people with disabilities on the sidelines cheering me and all of the other runners on."

The moral of the story and the lesson learned: In life, sometimes we see people who are better equipped to live life than we are. A person may write better or speak better, a person may be in better shape, more muscular or able to run better, a person may be able to sing better, but that doesn't mean that I cannot live a beautiful and happy life and enjoy what I have. Live life anyway. If you ever feel weak and want to give up, look at the finish line. There will always be others that are not as fortunate and they would be happy to trade places with us. God bless and stay safe.

– CHAPTER 6 –

THE ULTIMATE AND FINAL DECISION: POLICE OFFICERS AND SUICIDE

For the meaning of life differs from man to man, from day to day and from
hour to hour. What matters, therefore, is not the meaning of life in general
but rather the specific meaning of a person's life at a given moment.
Viktor Frankel

To run away from trouble is a form of cowardice and, while it is true that the
suicide braves death, he does it not for some noble object but to escape some ill.
Aristotle

ON FEBRUARY 27, 2020, Attorney General William P. Barr spoke at the International Association of Chiefs of Police Officer Safety and Wellness Symposium in Miami, Florida

> The rate of suicide among those in law enforcement and firefighting is 40 percent higher than the national average. Nearly one in four officers experience thoughts of suicide at some point in their lives. At least 228 officers took their own lives in 2019—a 44-percent increase from the previous year. Not only is that higher

than the number of line-of-duty deaths, it reflects a steady increase in officer suicides over the past several years.[7]

I believe that officers who take their lives have been constantly tormented in their struggles and issues to the point of ending it all. They've wrestled with their situation many times over, weighing the pros and cons as they contemplate life without them for the people they'll leave behind, wondering what kind of accident will dignify the loss of their life, rationalizing the scenario where everyone would be better if they were gone. Sure, they think, friends and family will grieve, but if I plan it just right it will look like an accident, not a suicide. Taking themselves out of the picture, they believe, will make things easier on everyone. It is sad to say, but to them it seems their best and only option at the time.

Police suicide is not just a problem—it is an epidemic. Yearly statistics indicate more police officers die by suicide than in line-of-duty deaths. Police culture, in my opinion, is the demoralizing culprit, major factor, and common denominator in most police suicides. Police suicide and the importance of police officers seeking emotional wellness are topics that are rarely brought up by law enforcement management, supervisors, or, for that matter, police officers themselves.

How disturbing is this remarkably common scenario? Bill is sitting at the kitchen table by himself with a half-empty bottle of whiskey and his service revolver next to him. He is crying because his wife has left him for good this time. They've fought about his drinking and verbal abuse, and now he's hit her one too many times. Bill has been a police officer for more than twenty-eight years, and he is nearing retirement. He is not well liked at work because he is always angry and irritated by everyone he works with. Bill's drinking has caused him to be late many times to roll call, and he was suspended for two days for insubordination and verbally abusing a citizen on his beat. He has no plans after his career is over. His life is in shambles. His mortgage is past due. Bill mumbles that he has nothing to live for as horrible and destructive thoughts race through his mind. He is in crisis and wondering if the pain will

---

[7] https://www.justice.gov/opa/speech/attorney-general-william-p-barr-delivers-remarks-international-association-chiefs-police

ever end. Now, with nowhere to turn and no light at the end of the tunnel, the disheartened officer's only alternative is to end the misery. Bill lifts his service revolver to his temple, and in a split second his emotional chaos is over.

A one-time wonderful, genuine, and caring officer took his own life when it could have all been worked out. Nothing is so hopeless that a solution cannot be found.

Retired Minnesota Peace Officer Duane Wolfe, who held positions as a patrolman, sergeant, special response team member, and a use-of-force and firearms instructor, almost didn't live long enough to begin his more-than twenty-five-year service career.

> I sat in my apartment alone, the room illuminated only by the light coming from the TV. I watched the changing colors dance across the satin blue finish as I opened the cylinder and loaded the .357.
>
> The past five years—one fifth of my life at age twenty-five—had all been wasted. I'd gone to college, gotten my degree, and even graduated as the "outstanding" Criminal Justice student.
>
> Yet jobs were tight, and despite my best efforts, I couldn't find a job no matter what I did.
>
> ### We Were Through
>
> She had made it tolerable by being there for me, and telling me that it was just a matter of time, and that things would work out.
>
> We were in love and had talked of marriage. We had problems in our five-year relationship, like every couple, but nothing that our love for each other couldn't overcome.
>
> Then she told me we were through.
>
> I tried to decide if I should put the muzzle in my mouth or press it against my temple. I would have loved to have picked up the phone and called my best friend. I had been the best man at his wedding. He was off doing what Army Rangers do, in undisclosed locations on confidential missions, and he wasn't taking calls.
>
> I had never been so alone.

I pressed the muzzle to my temple and cocked the hammer, my finger going to the trigger. I had no future.

"Give me one good reason why I shouldn't blow my brains out."

"There's always tomorrow."

I put the gun away and went to bed. I have been told that putting down that gun was an act of courage. I felt a great burden lifted off my shoulders and a resolve to never come to that point again.

I'd like to tell you that the next day the phone rang and she had changed her mind.

That call would never come.

I'd love to tell you that the next day the sun seemed to shine a little brighter and birds sang a little sweeter, but they didn't.

She Knew Too

The fact is, the next day sucked. Just like the days and weeks that followed, because unfortunately change never seems to happen as quickly as we would like it. But, I was alive to embrace the suck.

It wasn't easy but I kept plugging away at trying to find a job. I had given up on dating knowing that I could never love someone the way I loved her.

About three months later, I saw a face in a crowd, our eyes met and I knew.

She knew, too.

Two years later, (remember, things take time) we married and I became a police officer in the same week.

No, we didn't live happily ever after—that only happens in fairy tales. Life still hands us good and bad. We lost her dad to cancer. My wife's brother and my cousin would commit suicide.

There are the ups and downs of family, life, and profession. The good days far outweigh the bad ones. We have more excellent days than we are entitled to, and after almost thirty years, we still love each other a little more each day. So while it's no fairy-tale ending, it's pretty damn sweet. ...

I still have that gun. It was my first sidearm and I carried it on duty for years and it kept me safe and protected from harm. I kept it for that reason and because every time I see it, it is a reminder. "There's always tomorrow." [8]

When someone takes their own life, most people do not understand their reasoning. Family members and friends will be the first ones to blame themselves as they search for signs they did not catch or ignored if they did. Guilt is an extraordinary and destructive emotion. They ask themselves why they did not see the signs or do something sooner to prevent their loved one from taking their life.

Chaplain Mike Jones says,

As a chaplain, suicide has been a substantial part of what I do when it comes to notifying loved ones of the person who died. We assist the police in delivering probably the worst news a family will hear or experience in their lifetime. It could be their significant other, son, daughter, or another family member that has taken their life. It is not an easy message to deliver, and certainly not a good message to hear. It is absolutely devastating.

We try to comfort these people in the darkest hours of their lives, which is unimaginable unless a person has been there. Fortunately, I have never had to hear these words, but I have had there to say them numerous times; either way, it is very traumatic. It is hard knocking on a door at two am, waking someone up, knowing that when they see the police and a chaplain, they instantly know something terribly wrong has happened.

Every reaction to a death notification is different. A person hearing the news may often think if they had changed their behavior, had done or not done something differently, or said or not said something, their loved one would still be there. Their loved ones often blame themselves. It is not cause and effect. The

---

[8] https://www.police1.com/health-fitness/articles/the-day-i-put-a-gun-to-my-head-PoupY1KacQs28Au3/

loved ones need to know and understand that the decision someone makes to take their own life is their own; a loved one did not
make that decision for that person nor are they the cause of it. The
first reaction of many loved ones when notified about a suicide is
utter disbelief. They cling on any hope of mistaken identity and
that the loved one is still alive. Before we do our notifications,
we do our due diligence, making sure not only that we have the
correct person who has died but also the person we are speaking
with is the proper recipient of the news. It is important for us to
get the person notified to accept that their loved one is deceased
using the clear wording *has died*.

An officer's death is felt as a tremendous loss to their significant other,
parents, children, siblings, other relatives, friends, and acquaintances. The
officer's loss is also terribly painful among their police family; their partners,
fellow officers, supervisors, and citizens in their community. It also affects
the dispatcher who sends an officer to the scene who will make the initial
report, the paramedics who take the body away, and the detectives following
up and investigating the scene. That horrific scene is indelibly etched in the
memories of all who are dispatched. The person who takes their own life
destroys so many lives. The effect of suicide on a spouse or child is overwhelming; the hurt lasts forever and the grief and internal suffering never
go away. It is time for police suicide to be discussed openly and candidly
without fear of repercussion.

Jack A. Digliani, PhD, EdD, explains:

> The primary danger of policing has two components: one, phys-
> ical primary danger and two, psychological primary danger. The
> physical primary danger of policing is comprised of the inherent,
> potentially life-threatening risks of the job, such as working in
> motor vehicle traffic and confronting violent people. The psycho-
> logical primary danger of policing is represented in the increased
> probability that due to the nature of policing; officers will be
> exposed to critical incidents, work-related cumulative stress, and

human tragedy. This higher probability of exposure results in an increased likelihood that officers will suffer psychological traumatization and stressor-related disorders. Another way of saying this is that the physical primary danger of policing constitutes a work environment that generates the psychological primary danger of policing.

There is also an insidious and lesser-known secondary danger of policing, which is often unspecified and seldom discussed. It is an artifact of the police culture and is frequently reinforced by police officers themselves: It is the idea that equates "asking for help" with "personal and professional weakness." Secondary danger has been implicated in perhaps the most startling of all police fatality statistics, the frequency of police officer suicide.

Phil Epstein, MD, a Fulbright Scholar in neurochemistry, says,

Police constitute a separate and unique population, and in my opinion are at high risk of suicide because of the unusual intensity of the stress, the extent of the stress, and the unpredictability of the stress. These are all factors that can contribute to a person's self-assessment of being effective in their job. A person doesn't become a cop if they do not really believe that they are really making a difference. Law enforcement is always involving extremes of social behavior. They are dealing with individuals who exhibit erratic behavior, and these officers are at risk because of the dangerous behaviors they encounter. In general, these officers often are not talking to anyone about the issues they are experiencing. This puts officers at a greater potential risk for them to take their own lives.

Doug Monda, founder of Survive First, says,

Police suicide is rampant; it is getting worse and worse. The bottom line is that the law enforcement career is too much. It demands too much. What people forget is that cops are not robots, they are human beings. Human beings can only take so much pain before they shut down.

I have a metaphor for this: most cops are like an engine. Most people know how the basics of an engine and how an engine works. Take the biggest, meanest diesel engine on the planet; it's powerful and can run forever and ever. If a person takes a little bit of sand and drops it into the carburetor of that diesel engine, the first day not a big deal, the second day not a big deal. If a person continues to do that time and time again, what is going to happen to that diesel engine? After a while, the engine is going to seize up and quit running.

The diesel engine is more powerful than a human body. The metaphor of the story is this: If you think of the sand as the officer's trauma and the engine as the officer's brain, just like that engine, if you keep adding trauma, sooner or later that officer's brain is going to seize up. When it seizes up and doesn't want to work, it shuts down. Once it shuts down, there is nothing they can do about it, and that where the suicide comes in.

That is what happened to me. I consider myself an engine. I am a fifty-year-old guy who is in better shape than most guys in their thirties. I always ran at one hundred miles per hour and I'm highly physically, trained as an athlete. After a while the injuries came, the mental injuries and physical injuries came, and my body and mind could not take it anymore. I couldn't medicate the physical and mental pain and the only way my body and my mind could handle all that pain was to shut down. The only way to shut it down was to turn off the motor. For me, that was putting a gun to my head and pulling the trigger.

If we don't fix this problem now, it is only going to get worse. Ninety percent of cops working today have not experienced anything like we are experiencing right now with the coronavirus pandemic. Most generations experienced something tragic, like polio and smallpox, but this generation has never experienced anything like this COVID-19 era. It is traumatizing as officers are going to work with something else on their plates to deal with. Now they when have to get out of their squad, they're not only worrying about getting shot, but they have to worry about people breathing on them and making them sick. Then they worry about going home and giving it to their families.

If we do not train newer cops properly or change the way we do business, it is not going to work. It's going to get worse and worse and worse.

Police supervisors and patrolmen rarely discuss the subject of police suicide, not wanting to talk about the obvious elephant in the room. In every city throughout the country, police management does not want to embellish any police suicide. They want their citizens within their jurisdiction to know that the officers under their command are competent and well-adjusted to do their job.

SEEKING HELP

Police officers will often interject their own thoughts and feelings about the entire counseling system. If a police officer seeks psychological assistance at a mental hospital or facility or calls 911 indicating they have suicidal thoughts, their call is now on record. Most police jurisdictions will be notified that their officers have checked in for mental health reasons and/or evaluations and treatment. Many officers who seek treatment will always be worried that this may cost them their job in law enforcement. There are many officers who call out-of-state police suicide help lines just to ensure their confidentiality is preserved and their own police agency will not be alerted to their emotional well-being issues.

In Illinois, if an officer seeks help by entering a psychiatric hospital or facility, they will automatically have their FOID [Firearms Owners Identification] card taken away. In Illinois, police officers are required to carry a valid FOID card to work in law enforcement. Without a FOID card, that officer will not be able to carry a weapon, and therefore will be unable to work in law enforcement, and most likely not be able to work as a police officer ever again. At this point, the police officer seeking psychiatric help and support may be considered a liability for their department.

We need to support any officer requesting help without punishing them by taking away their law enforcement job or career. On August 26, 2018, former Illinois Governor Bruce Rauner signed into law House Bill 5231, which eliminated a job requirement that would temporarily revoke the Firearms Owners Identification card when an officer seeks mental health treatment. The move prevents police agencies from requiring a FOID card as a condition of continued employment. Illinois law now allows police officers to seek mental health treatment without fear of losing their jobs, though there is a stipulation that an officer would still have their FOID card taken away if they are deemed to be a threat to themselves or others and deemed unfit for duty.

RELIEVING AN OFFICER OF THEIR DUTIES

It is obvious that relieving an officer of their duties will have a domino effect. They have a family to support—a mortgage, car payment, or tuition. With that source of income gone, if the same officer is already in despair, they may become even more depressed. An officer is built up to be brave, strong, and unbreakable, but as human beings we have breaking points. As humans, we have feelings—we do get angry and, most of all, we unload and let go of our emotional baggage.

The consequence is that an officer who sought out help or treatment from anyone in the mental health field could possibly lose their job because of their situation. Who would hire them with this red flag on their record? The chance of suicide becomes even greater. With nowhere to turn and no solution in sight, the disheartened officer may use their own service weapon as the only alternative to ease the pain.

SUICIDE "IN THE LINE OF DUTY"

An officer who is emotionally lost and desperate will often look for ways that will make their intentional death appear to be an accident, or in a way that makes them look like a hero. In their mind, they have decided they want to die, so why not go out a hero instead of someone who is weak? They may be or are thinking, "What a great way to end it all, receive a hero's burial as an officer killed in the line of duty and my family is compensated because of my death."

These officers look for ways to be the first to go through a barricaded door while serving a warrant. Who would argue against their actions constituting bravery as they act with little or no regard for their own safety? When they rarely step back and wait for assistance? In some police academies, they call this the *John Wayne Syndrome*, which is related to the attitude of "I can do it all" that may ultimately get that officer seriously hurt or killed.

The official report may read that the officer was cleaning his duty weapon when it accidentally discharged. The assertion concludes the officer died by a gun cleaning accident, not by suicide. By labeling the death something other than a suicide, the officer's reputation and action would not shame their family or the department and the officer's family would be able to collect his/her unclaimed benefits.

Chaplain Al Lopez, of the Chicago Police Department, says,

> Police suicide is a silent illness. The person with this illness often does not reveal or share it with anyone. They often have a difficult time reaching out regarding what issues they are having. It is a constant and endless fight because they often struggle with torment as they search for a way out from what is bothering them. I suggest they pursue spiritual guidance and seek out the Lord, who made a promise never to abandon us no matter what we are going through.

Dr. Frank Campbell, founder of Local Outreach of Suicide Survivors (LOSS), says,

A police officer is five times more likely to use their service revolver on themselves than to kill an offender. The aftermath of suicide has an effect on the human mind. Training law enforcement in suicide prevention is imperative. We know it works. The concept is similar to a person drowning. If we train everyone to be a lifeguard, we will have fewer people drown.

Luke Fairless, PsyD, a clinical psychologist employed with the Illinois Department of Corrections, noted that recent research from the Michigan Department of Corrections shows a copious number of suicides in the past few years.

The Michigan Department of Corrections brought in a few experts who found that almost every state experienced a rise in correctional suicide. [Combine] inmates with mental illness and the rising tide of stress in law enforcement, and we are seeing a perfect storm. In the last five years, suicide rates in rural areas has increased among white male correctional officers that the Department of Corrections employs.

We are trying to collect data on trends to better prevent suicide and to fine tune our responses to help our correctional officers. Even one suicide is too many!

Police deal with the worst of humanity on a daily basis, Trying to deal with traumatic incidents and trying to process what they experience is difficult. These officers have to try to maintain a proper outlook with society and themselves. Officers are worried about things in their career that have gone wrong or they know that they done wrong, allegations of misconduct, and how to deal with the consequences. Some officers see suicide as the only way out. We have been in situations like that where we have to tell a husband or wife that their loved one is gone. Helping the loved one establish a support group is important in getting out of that denial phase. Everyone has their own level of how they process suicide of a loved one.

We try to help officers on our end with resiliency seminars. These seminars help officers understand their emotions. Our seminars do not single out officer's specific individual problems in open, public format where police are concerned. Police are unlikely to deal with personal issues in public, particularly in a setting with their fellow officers in attendance.

Chaplain Jones has held debriefings where many officers were open to issues regarding traumatic events they've encountered include shootings, an officer being shot or injured, where an officer had to take someone's life in the course of duty, or an officer's child who took their own life. When an officer is in a debriefing situation like that, sharing with other officers may help in the healing process.

Father Dan Brandt, director of the Chicago Police Chaplain's Unit, agrees.

We have our share of issues. In 2018, we lost four officers in the line of duty, and nine officers, including retirees who died of suicide. In 2019, we had six officers die of suicide. I am fearing it is going to be another tough year with all that is going on in today's society. The hatred that is out there from the mayor, the county board, the politicians, to the misguided and uneducated loud mouths who do not support our officers. These officers are constantly hearing that they are no good from everyone, and sooner or later they are going to start believing it.

Chaplain Jones believes officers want to take a problem and fix it, but many of these problems are not so easily fixed.

Officers put a tremendous burden on themselves trying to heal from what may take years to heal from. Officers need to learn to be available for their fellow officers, not just for two or three weeks but for the long haul. it is important that the officer does not retreat into self-medication such as alcohol or drugs or unhealthy or toxic behavior that will hurt them immediately or down the road. It is important for officers to know what to do if one of their fellow officers need help. It is OK to be human; they don't have to fix the problem immediately but just be there if they are needed.

There is no immediate fix for some of these horrific situations they may not be able to handle by themselves. It is important for them to seek references, therapists, or counselors for a myriad of support. We live in the land between the brave and the broken, trying to keep the brave from being broken, and trying to help the broken be brave. There is that land and the land we live in.

Dr. Olivia Johnson, founder of the Blue Wall Institute, agrees that suicide among law enforcement personnel is not a new phenomenon. Rather, this threat is receiving the attention it rightfully deserves ... but not by viewing each suicide as a statistic.

Numbers are being thrown out that cannot be verified. It has even been suggested that officer deaths deemed "unexpected" and "sudden" are included in these suicide numbers without proper verification. In some venues, these men and women are seen as no more than a number. They become marginalized and then sensationalized with little being done to stop this threat. True research must be done. Our law enforcement professionals deserve better.

Suicide is not easily explained or understood by those lacking the appropriate background and experience to do so. For example, while there are cases in which PTSD will have a significant impact, trying to say that the majority of cases are PTSD-related is irresponsible and does not accurately reflect this multidimensional phenomenon.

We also know that stress and the inability to deal with personal and professional stressors appropriately plays a significant role. We have men and women under extreme amounts of stress just from the job, including trauma, critical incidents, and departmental strife. Then we have these officers going home unable to address or handle these experiences positively. Many will never receive the true degree of professional assistance needed to maintain a healthy work-life balance. This in turn can lead to relationship issues such as divorce, separation, or break-ups, physical and mental health issues, disciplinary issues, early retirement, job loss, and substance abuse issues.. The cycle will continue unless broken, often with negative results such a suicide.

Police psychologist Dr. Marla Friedman says,

The only consistent variable that I can identify and occurs in every suicide is pain. Physical or emotional pain. Continued research is needed to fully comprehend the act of suicide within law enforcement and other first responders as well as the general population.

The number one issue continues to be the stigma related to seeking and maintaining good mental health. Law enforcement culture continues to support the concept that asking for help is a weakness. Utilizing therapy or peer support services is also interpreted as a risk to career advancement. In reality, a mentally and physically healthy officer is more efficient, alert, compassionate, at ease with themselves will be able to attend to what is happening in the environment. The result is decreased use of force complaints, decreased implicit bias (correlated to sleep shift disorder), less alcoholism, fewer divorces, decreased grievances filed against the department, fewer officers calling off sick, and increased satisfaction and safety for the officer, their family and the public.

It must start at the top with every police department, where police chiefs agree to visit a mental health professional, showing those under their command that it is acceptable to seek mental health. Officers are not going to risk taking that first step to health without a support safety net from management.

Each department knows how many suicides they have. Most police administrations want the public to believe they address the emotional needs of their officers. Typically, they don't want the information to leave the department. Officers who take their own lives are often not honored for their prior service, their funerals are private, and a few members from their own departments attend. From that point forward they are rarely mentioned, and they become ghosts and are soon forgotten. More recently, some departments are starting to be more open about police suicide and acknowledge their devastating loss. That is when they start searching for reasons and seeking programming that will educate their officers. An after-action review should be mandatory following a suicide, for many reasons. One suicide gives permission for another person who has been thinking about it. Suicide is contagious. Departments need a plan as to how to manage the thoughts and feelings of survivors. Compilation of data may help illuminate the reasons the officer chose suicide. Sometimes suicides are directly related to something that happened on the job or reasons that are totally unrelated. There is a tremendous amount of work to be done in this area.

Blue Wall Institute founder Dr. Olivia Johnson believes the answer lies in proactive and readily available assistance for officers and their families.

Officers must receive the information and resources to help facilitate the healthy work-life balance before issues arise. It is important that they never have to go looking for help. Finding help in crisis is not how the system is supposed to work. Seeking assistance should not be punitive. Of course there will be times when officers will not be deemed "fit for duty," but this should be the exception, not the rule.

Agency leaders must set the example of seeking assistance, which is beneficial in many ways. If an officer has a crisis or experiences a critical incident, seeking professional assistance in a timely manner is critical. It does not have to be through the officer's agency. We have many organizations these officers can call for help and remain confidential. Officers must be aware of numerous resources, not just those provided by their agency. Agency leaders should spend time not only seeking out organizations that may be beneficial, but making phone calls and finding out what happens when an officer calls in. What steps will they go through? What should they expect?

Having the employee assistance program is not enough. Many officers do not trust agency-affiliated organizations. We know this and must do more than just say we are providing something. One of the largest hurdles is not knowing what is available and what rights the officer has. They need to know what happens when they reach out. Step by step. No surprises. The biggest thing that keeps officers from seeking assistance is fear. Fear of the unknown. Fear should never be a hurdle to being well. Let's work together to tear down these hurdles and help this nation's officer receive the help they so rightly deserve.

EMPLOYEE ASSISTANCE PROGRAMS

We need to support any officer requesting help without punishing them by taking away their job or career. An officer's law enforcement position may be the only source of income for their family. An officer should not have to deal with the emotional trauma from the stress of the job, the stress from family life, and the stress from management.

Dr. Jack Digliani says the availability of an employee assistance program, or EAP, and insurance plan community counseling services for police officers represents a significant advancement in the delivery of counseling services. He believes they are helpful in that they are utilized by some officers who might not otherwise seek assistance. However, although helpful, EAPs and health plan counseling appear insufficient. Despite their availability, they do not and cannot meet the needs of many police officers.

The Chicago Police Department, like those in many other large cities, has an excellent Employee Assistance Program that deals with officers who may be experiencing emotional difficulties, either personal or job-related. The only problem with the Chicago EAP Unit is that it is understaffed. There have been only three full-time clinicians for 13,500 officers for many years. In Los Angeles, there are twelve full-time clinicians for 10,000 officers. Just recently, Chicago has brought on six more clinicians to their EAP staff.

SEEKING HELP IS NOT A SIGN OF WEAKNESS

Vickie Poklop, a police counselor with the Des Plaines, Illinois Police Department, suggests that talking to a counselor or a therapist doesn't have to be scary.

> [Asking for help] is not a sign of weakness. It is a sign or strength to ask someone for a helping hand. I view therapy as a collaboration between therapist and client. The client gets to decide what to talk about, what to work on, what direction to go in the sessions. The client has self-determination to decide what needs addressing now and what can wait until later. A therapist's job is to provide healing for the part of the client that isn't feeling so well. Healing comes from talk therapy, hypnotherapy, and many other kinds of therapies that can be used during a session. Healing comes in layers, which is why it feels so good to release all the unnecessary baggage that holds us down and back. Whether they are officers or not, I always say to all my clients, "We all need helpers to get through this crazy life. Nobody gets through this life alone." How could a person possibly navigate living a life all by themselves, without any outside help, without any outside advice, without any outside intervention, without a compassionate ear and a tear catcher, how would they do it? How would they do it without their friends and their families and the people they trust?

The Dane Smith Story: A Tragic Ending to a Young Police Officer's Life

Officer Dane Smith took his own life using his duty weapon in the early morning hours, on the frigid morning of January 1, 2019. Dane was a family man who loved his wife, Nicole, and his young son. It was difficult for everyone who knew him to accept the fact that he took his own life. His suicide had a ripple effect of sadness, grief, and other emotions for everyone who knew and worked with this young Chicago Police officer.

Chicago Police Sergeant Jeff Sachs, Dane's stepdad, who raised Officer Smith since he was a young boy, shares his story.

> Dane battled depression the last few years of his life. He joined the Chicago Police Department after serving his country in the United States Army. My stepson was athletic and recently competed in a rival boxing match between the Chicago Police Department and the Chicago Fire Department in the *Battle of the Badges*. Dane won the bout in his weight class. He was a tough kid, and he had no problem working in the Englewood district, one of the most dangerous districts in the city, noted for its high rate of crime and homicides. I believe that the police culture combined with constantly working in that environment took its toll on Dane and on his marriage. He soon started drinking with his fellow officers after work.
>
> One night after getting drunk in the fall of 2017, Dane threatened suicide. The Chicago Police employee assistance program (EAP) unit was summoned because Dane was worried that the State Police would take his FOID card, preventing him from being a police officer. He soon went to see a professional clinician to discuss the issues that were plaguing him. Dane seemed better after that, but he kept drinking to drown his sorrows.

Dane's brother, Jon, believes the police culture was to blame for his excessive drinking.

> Dane was never like this before. Dane asked to be transferred to headquarters, as he thought a change would do him good. After

another drunken episode, Dane came home and aggressively told his wife to leave the house. Nicole left with their son and stayed with her family. They soon separated because Nicole asked for a divorce.

Dane's stepfather continued:

The excessive drinking was just the tip of the iceberg. Pending divorce, prescription drugs, he was overextended with his credit, often living higher than his means, the culmination of drinking, stress of the job, a new and rocky marriage, new house, not wanting to be with his extended family (he became a loner) and pressure about finances (debtors calling often), and not paying back his brother, who cosigned for his car loan led to his demise.

On New Year's Eve, Dane called his brother Jon to go out and celebrate. Jon regretfully declined because he was not feeling well. By himself, and depressed after another night of excessive drinking, Dane took his life, believing that his life was not worth anything. I was shocked to hear the news and was in disbelief, and dismayed that I hadn't done more as guilt filled my heart and soul.

Sachs had guilt as a father over not doing more for his stepson, for not being a pest in Dane's life or staying in better communication with Dane. Sachs admitted Dane would never have killed himself had he not been drunk. Leading up to New Year's Eve, it was the perfect storm which no one saw coming.

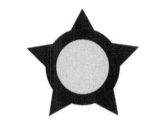

PART TWO

FINDING A SOLUTION

– CHAPTER 7 –

THE IMPORTANCE OF MENTAL HEALTH TREATMENT

Constant kindness can accomplish much. As the sun makes ice melt,
kindness causes misunderstanding, mistrust, and hostility to evaporate.
Albert Schweitzer

IT IS AMAZING how resilient police officers are at handling the problems they face and their daily stressors. Since I began writing this book, our nation has experienced hundreds of thousands of deaths from the COVID-19 virus, as well as a loss of jobs, and a struggling economy. To add fuel to the fire, we are experiencing a hatred for the police that I have never seen before. There has been a recent escalation of peaceful and violent protesting, looting, arson, and criminal damage to property triggered by poor judgment in the arrest and death of a career criminal named George Floyd, Brianna Taylor, and others.

Many media-sensationalized situations that involve police shooting across the county have fanned the flames of hatred for law enforcement. The stress felt by police officers has increased tenfold. Making matters worse, many departments have their officers working twelve-hour shifts with few or no days off for extended periods of time and communities are calling to defund police departments across the United States. There is a general disregard for law enforcement by many in every city throughout America. Officers are tired mentally, physically, and emotionally, yet they persevere day in and day out as they are pushed to their limits. Some people are coping with it; others are having a difficult time. Seeking mental health support can be an invaluable tool in helping officers cope with everything they deal with on the job.

Thayer Crouse, Director of Development and Outreach for the Chateau Recovery Treatment Center in Midway, Utah, is often frustrated by the uphill battle his agency fights to help officers receive mental health treatment.

> We are finding that management in many police agencies are worried about liability for officers seeking mental health treatment. We are trying to get across to numerous police administrations that it is more cost effective to invest in an officer seeking mental health treatment. Providing mental health treatment to an experienced officer is a fraction of the cost of training a new officer. A first responder who has sought treatment will be a better officer, father, or mother. Why would that administration not want to support that? There are still a lot of police departments that are seeing the logic of getting their officer well again, but there are still a number of departments who are not investing money in their officers who are struggling with emotional issues.

Denise M. Coyle, LMFT, CTS, has witnessed the importance of command support.

> One of the things the Drug Enforcement Administration (DEA) has done really well is address cultural issues. They have made it so that mental health is incorporated in what they do with their trauma teams. We, the mental health professionals, do not take over a scene (critical incident), but we support the scene. We support the peer groups, and we are there, sort of like an escalation. Peer support keeps us in the loop, and we assist them. If a higher level of care is needed, then and only then do we step in. Even

then, we utilize the peer support team throughout. What I have discovered in working with some of the police departments is this: if management and the change of command is supportive, officers have a higher success rate in returning to duty. They also have a higher success rate in decreasing how many officers develop post-traumatic stress disorder (PTSD). The command supports through their creation of a structure that not only acknowledges the potential for trauma and stress but also implements a plan to support those with the courage to speak up and seek help.

I had an officer who was sent to me who was put on leave for thirty days to get treatment for post-traumatic stress. The command staff was phenomenal. Whatever the person needed; if he needed time, he was given time; if he needed a peer, he was given a peer, etc. They checked in on him, and they were supportive. When the officer returned to duty, everyone was completely on board. It started these conversations among the members of the department about what they had struggled with and what they needed. This actually led to a bigger peer support team and to the officer giving a presentation on the impact of trauma and seeking services with complete command support.

The biggest change in culture is not only from the bottom up, but actually from the top down. When officers know they are truly supported by management, they do not have a problem asking for help. The other aspect is normalizing and talking about critical incidences that they have experienced. Everyone thinks there has to be a hardline Critical Incident Stress Management (CISM) that centers on a direct and recognizable problem. When management encourages and wants to talk about "what just happened," there is such a huge benefit. Talking about the incident right away, but not necessarily making it a CISM call. There has to be degrees of intervention. When there is a bad situation, just talk about it: What happened? What do you think? What are you feeling? Check in and make having a conversation about an event become normal. There should be somebody, whether it is peer support, a chaplain, or mental health person there to do a check-in. "I heard you had a pretty rough call, what is going on?" Make that a normal part of any call that involves a death, or when an officer comes upon a body, or something that would be considered a significant trauma. If we can start talking about traumatic situations and our reactions to them, we normalize them, and then they becomes easier to process. When an officer feels like they can't say anything because they have to be tough or because nobody is talking about it, then the trauma becomes detrimental. Having peer support get involved, "I heard the last shift had a critical incident, I am here to do a post check," that would be ideal.

INTERNAL FAMILY SYSTEMS THERAPY (IFST)

The Internal Family Systems Therapy model, created and developed by Dr. Richard Schwartz, combines "the complex external family system" with the view that "individuals are composed of separate and multifaceted internal parts in relationship with each other."

Four Elements of the Internal Family Systems Therapy Model
Sonja DePratt is a licensed clinical social worker with over twenty years of experience who often incorporates the IFST method in her therapy sessions. Many of her patients are law enforcement personnel struggling with an enormous amount of stress and personal issues, as well as PTSD.

"The Internal Family Systems Therapy," DePratt explains, "has four basic elements associated with humanity, and all are interactive with each other. All four aspects of IFST model of humanness are involved in any situation, both positive and negative."

Biological. DePratt reminds us that the physical body is affected by stress and the many stressors we endure.

Our bodies are fully engaged in the moment, dominated by the situation. The more a person's awareness level increases, the more resilient they become. The more people take care of their bodies the more their awareness increases. Honoring a person's body through proper diet exercise and rest will also keep that person emotionally well.

Psychological (mind and emotion). DePratt explains how the psychological aspects of being human affect a person's thoughts, beliefs, emotions, and their conscious and subconscious mind.

Different areas of the mind get engaged for various reasons. The more self-aware we are of our internal dynamics, the more we can develop the ability and skills to regulate our emotional reactions. A person's emotional reactions create a greater clarity and awareness of the big picture. If police officers can calm down their internal trigger, then they can open up more transparency and understanding within themselves.

DePratt gives a good example of what almost every police officer encounters on a daily basis, and that is anger. "Anger often hijacks an officer's emotions as their vision narrows—they literally only see the target of what got them angry. If that officer could only step back and calm down and reaccess the situation, they are more likely to see the big picture and react differently."

Social. DePratt says the third aspect of understanding a person's social environment is to see how they are affected by that environment.

Everyone is impacted by how they were raised, the culture they know and cherish, and how that individual sees the situation through their own experience. As we are all different, we have insight and awareness as we try to understand the perspective of others. If a person came from a racist home, they will more likely be impacted by racial issues and have a greater response to the many different races they encounter throughout their life. Everyone experiences cultural prejudices. Awareness of these cultural prejudices helps a person become more objective of what they see and how well they deal with the situation. Understanding the impact of every aspect of our experiences helps us to evaluate the accuracy and validity of our beliefs and our understanding of ourselves.

Our reactions are often directly tied to a belief we have internalized as children. Children pick up the burden of this viciousness early in their life. For example, when a young five-year-old is constantly told they are stupid and will never amount to anything. This message is absorbed internally, and they begin to believe that they are really stupid. If that young person never evaluates that "burden," they may react negatively to "stupid" when they hear it, and that same hurt resurfaces and again they become traumatized.

Spiritual. When a police officer witnesses evil or trauma, says DePratt, they may react with a crisis of faith.

This continuous trauma often results in PTSD. It is not uncommon for police officers, like soldiers, to experience the reoccurring tragedies they have experienced throughout their careers. That police officer's faith is often questioned; as it leaves a mark on their soul. Police officers may question their very existence as they continuously experience inhumane tragedy on a day-to-day basis. A police officer may ask themselves, "Why am I here? What is the mission in my life?"

ELEMENTS OF THE "MAKE IT SAFE" POLICE OFFICER INITIATIVE

Jack A. Digliani, PhD, EdD, creator of the "Make It Safe" Police Officer Initiative, explains that the twelve elements of the Initiative are designed to reduce the secondary danger of policing and, thereby, police officer suicide. The Make It Safe Initiative Police Officer Initiative encourages:

1. every officer to "self-monitor" and to take personal responsibility for his or her mental wellness.
2. every officer to seek psychological support when confronting potentially overwhelming difficulties (officers do not have to go it alone).
3. every officer to diminish the sometimes deadly effects of secondary danger by reaching out to other officers known to be facing difficult circumstances.
4. veteran and ranking officers to use their status to help reduce secondary danger (veteran and ranking officers can reduce secondary danger by openly discussing it, appropriately sharing selected personal experiences, avoiding the use of pejorative terms to describe officers seeking or engaging psychological support, and talking about the acceptability of seeking psychological support when confronting stressful circumstances.
5. law enforcement administrators to better educate themselves about the nature of secondary danger and to take the lead in secondary danger reduction.
6. law enforcement administrators to issue a departmental memo encouraging officers to engage psychological support services when confronting potentially overwhelming stress (the memo should include information about confidentiality and available support resources).
7. basic training in stress management, stress inoculation, critical incidents, post-traumatic stress, police family dynamics, substance use and addiction, and the warning signs of depression and suicide.
8. the development of programs that engage preemptive, early-warning, and periodic department-wide officer support interventions (for

example, proactive annual check in, "early warning" policies designed to support officers displaying signs of stress, and regularly scheduled stress inoculation and critical incident stressor management training).

9.   law enforcement agencies to initiate incident-specific protocols to support officers and their families when officers are involved in critical incidents.

10. law enforcement agencies to create appropriately structured, properly trained, and clinically supervised peer support teams.

11. law enforcement agencies to provide easy and confidential access to counseling and specialized police psychological support services.

12. police officers at all levels of the organization to enhance the agency climate so that others are encouraged to ask for help when experiencing psychological or emotional difficulties instead of keeping and acting out a deadly secret.

Denise Coyle, LMFT, CTS, sums it up this way:

> One difficult realization for an officer to accept and come to terms with is the idea that they need psychological help. This needed assistance could be from previous incidents in the first responder's childhood or from trauma-related to incidents that they have experienced on the job. The hardest decision they will ever have to make is accepting help and therapy that they never thought they needed. Seeking treatment will ultimately be the best decision they will ever make if they want to live an emotionally happy life.

– CHAPTER 8 –

CHATEAU RECOVERY: A DIFFERENT TREATMENT APPROACH

*Our job on earth isn't to criticize, reject, or judge. Our purpose
is to offer a helping hand, compassion and mercy. We are to
do unto others as we hope they would do onto us.*
Dana Acuri

CHATEAU RECOVERY IS A UNIQUE PROGRAM that specializes in helping individuals and families in various forms of crisis and offers different forms of recovery. The social definition of recovery used to be limited to only those struggling with substance and/or alcohol abuse, and traditional rehabs have been providing specific and targeted forms of treatment and support over the last seventy years. Even today, most treatment programs focus exclusively on substance abuse and helping people find abstinence from their drug of choice. Once they obtain abstinence, they are *in recovery* and need to maintain this status. This definition used to be the only way of measuring success in recovery. Chateau Recovery is interested in a broader understanding of recovery that is not limited to substance abuse alone but is focused on helping individuals "recover," heal, and grow in all dimensions of life.

This chapter is devoted to Chateau Recovery because Ben Pearson, Thayer Couse, and their entire team are well-known and dedicated in their confidential treatment for all first responders. The Chateau Recovery team is instrumental in designing specific treatment plans to help them tackle any issues they have encountered in their roles as first responders. They will help all first responders become a viable asset to their families and to their law enforcement communities once again.

Ben Pearson, LCSW, Chateau Recovery's clinical director, says,

> Our program is uniquely designed to help first responders and others rebuild their lives. The overall philosophy of the program is to undo the stigma around getting help, effectively address trauma, and provide an experience for first responders and others that is empowering and responsive to their individual needs. On top of being an innovative dual-diagnosis program, Chateau Recovery is focused on tackling the unique cultural challenges that responders and public safety agencies face.
>
> Police, firefighters, military, correctional officers, dispatchers, and other emergency medical services workers have their own unique cultures and personalities that are different throughout the country. When I speak about first-responder culture, I'm talking about the larger culture, and it's not always accurate to each individual or branch of responders. Within the larger culture, first responders have their own unique subculture that has significant strengths and challenges. The strengths include the heroic skills, logistical communication, team coordination, and professionalism that is frequently highlighted in movies and social media. These skills accompany a unique, service-oriented mindset that allows responders to run toward danger and face fears and challenges that would shut down the average person.
>
> One of the great upsides of working with first responders in treatment is that they typically have an awesome work ethic and can be focused and effective when their heads are clear of substances. When they are in this state, they are internally motivated to get to work on improving most aspects of their lives. In health, they are great at giving feedback, learning more effective

tools, and wanting to learn how to improve relationships as well as mindset. They come with a set of developed insights and tools that translate to self-care and self-improvement. These and other positive components of the responder culture should be supported, praised, and honored.

However, there are other aspects of the responder culture that do not get the kind of attention and support needed. This allows bad habits, toxic beliefs, and learned negative traditions to grow in the shadows and into broad daylight. The mental impact on a first responder who has experienced trauma and then quickly re-engages in emotionally demanding working conditions is often unnoticed and thus unaddressed by untrained supervisors, colleagues, and bystanders alike. Unfortunately, this can mean friends, family members, and others close to a responder do not see emotional barriers that can be crushing to the responder. The impact of stress on our responders is enormous. Unfortunately, these things are often hard for anyone to notice when our larger popular culture struggles to deal with or even talk about stress and mental health issues. Rarely does anyone get the kind of training required to deal with these issues for themselves or to offer effective help to another in need. Thus, responders are at an increased disadvantage when dealing with stress and trauma at work and at home.

Pearson goes on to talk about how our larger first responder culture struggles with stress.

A typical first responder or average person is under the impression they are not supposed to have stress in their life. Our cultural definition of happiness often includes the absence of stress or challenges. Not only is that assumption completely unrealistic, but it creates an unhealthy expectation around a normal emotion. Instead of learning to accept that stress plays an important role in our lives, we go the other direction. When this happens, we develop a distorted perspective and shame-based opinion about our stress. We begin to believe that something is wrong with us if we feel or connect with stress. This distorted mentality around not having stress has connections to a rise in depression and anxiety in our larger culture. The corporate and marketing world thrives on a culture that is terrified of experiencing stress and is constantly selling products and concepts that help us avoid feeling and coping with it.

As a whole, our culture is obsessed with getting rid of negative feelings like stress. It's not a coincidence that cigarettes, alcohol, sex and pornography, high-power toys, gambling, and other distractions are part of a billion-dollar industry that benefits from a culture that is overwhelmed and tired because they are in fear of feeling. It is also not a coincidence that responders lean heavily on these coping mechanisms to make it through the average week.

Like others, responders grow up in this culture of fear and learn these unrealistic expectations, emotions, and coping methods. They are not given adequate warning that these dangerous methods of managing stress and resisting it have devastating consequences. Ironically, they assume dependent or addictive thinking and self-medicating only applies to illicit drugs and irresponsible alcohol use. Recently, more camouflaged options like sugar, caffeine, over-the-counter medications, smoking, and energy drinks have become legal, socially acceptable, and readily available resources to remedy unwanted thoughts, fatigue, and social pressure. These substances and behaviors are designed to alter reality, enhance social performance, and reduce stress. Unbeknownst to the individual, however, when applying these false remedies, officers become stretched thinner mentally, develop shame around their emotions, and struggle even more to find and access healthy ways to express emotions and ask for help. Their families struggle to understand them and their burdens and watch powerlessly as their loved one is crushed by unexpressed emotions, negativity, resentment, undiagnosed depression, and PTSD.

To be clear, there is a lot of support, loyalty, and devotion that drives this culture. The brother and sisterhood of responders and veterans is powerful and is often the glue that keeps them continuing to work and give so much. Families of responders are known for their devotion and the enormous sacrifices they make to support their loved ones in providing these vital public services. However, there are some behaviors and traditions that are common within the responder culture that make healing from trauma more elusive and challenging. When it comes to substance recovery and/or getting mental and emotional help, individual responders and agencies often have tunnel vision around these problems and are unaware of how they spread. They often don't see the medical reality of how neglected issues are toxic and spread in the mind and body. Thus, they often have superficial assumptions around quick fixes and getting healthy.

When people subscribe to these popular but distorted assumptions around getting better and place their trust in this broken idea, they get hurt. This is why many people do not have hope or trust in the idea of getting help or finding treatment. One of the goals of Chateau Recovery is to help people see that recovery and treatment is a larger and more personal process than they anticipated. Our program is not about managing symptoms. It's about becoming and being a healthy person. It is not just controlling the use of a substance or monitoring the consequences of PTSD. That is a tunnel vision way of thinking about health. Thus, our biggest challenge is to help people shift how they think about getting help and staying healthy. People are unique, and each person struggles with individual challenges. Recovery is a challenging and empowering process of rediscovery and rebuilding to a better and more authentic version of ourselves.

This is why we challenge our staff and clients to think about the larger picture. We believe that all people, in general, are dynamic. They have multiple dimensions within themselves.

When we look at healing, we look at six different dimensions of wellness that include mental and emotional health, physical health, family systems, spirituality, personal/social relationships, and basic adult living skills. The purpose of the program is to help clients be as healthy as possible in each of the six dimensions of their life. Our goal is to help our client become more aware, accepting, and creative in problem-solving in each of the six dimensions. We believe a person can become healthier in each of these areas, then when challenged with stress and traumatic situations, clients will have a mental health cushion to rely on.

Previously, some clients had such high expectations of themselves or such rigid thinking that one bad day sends them over an edge. That can look like lapsing back into alcohol or substance abuse, or poor decisions that may cost the first responder their job or marriage. Many responders need help making this mental adjustment to self-care because they are often comfortable with rigidity and black-and-white problem-solving. Responders are often nervous initially as they are asked to consider this mindset shift and a new approach to being healthy. However, when they compare their old system with this newer model, they see that it makes sense on many levels.

THREE PILLARS OF THE CHATEAU RECOVERY PROGRAM

As mentioned previously, the Chateau is a unique program that is not trying to be like other facilities. We stay far away from the one-size-fits-all attitude about recovery and treatment as we support clients in healing, growing, and gaining new skills through the following three pillars of the program.

Whole Self: This means accepting, exploring, and treating all six dimensions of your whole self. It also means helping each individual understand their unique development, needs, and resources while preparing for the journey forward.

Mindset: This is about focusing energy on developing a healthy, empowered, and outward-focused mindset. Clients work toward a mindset that accepts difficulty and imperfection in themselves and in others. Each person is engaged in and responsible for building the best version of him or herself.

Resilience: This principle is about developing a resilient and healthy relationship with stress and change. It's not only improving skills but also refocusing time and effort into personal values and maintaining the course when faced with unexpected pain and trauma.

Pearson repeatedly made a strong and clear point that individuals, families, communities, and professionals need to compare and assume less and consider the uniqueness of each individual.

> Accepting and working with the quirks and strengths of each individual will always be the superior path to healing and reconnection. Getting away from formulas that require others to conform and perform lead to superficial—or sometimes dishonest—personal growth. Changing the expectation from behavior improvement to healing the deeper mindset requires a paradigm shift for everyone involved. Altering mindset is another level of self-improvement. Shifting perspective around our notions about change, growth, personal worth, and safety is some of the most important work we ever do as humans. It's deeply personal and requires a willingness and vulnerability that most people are often too intimidated to tackle.
>
> Although challenging, each person owning and championing this process is their responsibility and opportunity. Each of us needs to break the toxic dependence on formulas and assumptions that have been created over the years. Just like each of us digests and metabolizes substances differently, mindset change and personal growth function the same way. At Chateau, we have our clients look at themselves as unique individuals. They will soon find out that someone else's plan won't work for them. Thus, clients learn the importance of ownership, communication, and reliance on their individual programs to deal with stress and

trauma. Clients realize their motivations and solutions are unique for their own emotional wellness.

A first responder can borrow ideas and a handful of tools they have acquired from watching what has worked for others. This may be beneficial for a few weeks, or even a few months, but unless they create their own mindset, skills, and resources, their own individual path and plan, they will likely abandon their efforts and revert back to what is comfortable to them as soon as something falls apart. Our focus is on how we help clients encounter skills they believe in and take ownership of. That way, when bad days come, they know what works for them and are invested in their own healing. Taking ownership is not just a therapeutic gimmick, but a solution that is intended to become a lifestyle.

Beyond the ownership mentality, the program applies specific mindset tools developed by the Arbinger Institute. The Arbinger Institute has created a philosophy that helps individuals and corporations move beyond self-interest and reactive problem-solving. The emphasis on this dimension relies on interpersonal skills and social wellness. The Arbinger Institute deals with a person's outward mindset, which is basically to comprehend and understand others. This is an important and crucial portion of therapy. They teach that all people make a fundamental choice between seeing people as people or seeing them as objects. He explained that when we see people as objects, it changes our behaviors and thinking toward them. We tend to see them as threats, challenges, or barriers, or irrelevant to our personal goals and happiness. Unfortunately, when we see others like this, we justify our mistreatment of them and distort our vision of them and ourselves in the process. Instead of connecting, serving, and communicating effectively with them, we put on our mental armor and are resistant to their ideas and needs. The Chateau program helps responders and others transition back to a mindset that helps us humanize and regard others as people.

As individuals transform their mindset, they have less need for interpersonal defensiveness, manipulation, and isolation from relationships. They can start to approach themselves and others with more compassion, equality, and patience while looking for opportunities to find common solutions. This is a big deal when it comes to first responders. Many of them, after years of responding to horrible situations and needing to depersonalize situations and people to get the job done, find themselves in a mindset that is not the same as when they started the profession. That is why we see a lot of compassion fatigue, burnout, stress, depression, and anxiety among first responders. To protect themselves from a world that is full of threats, they typically and unconsciously go to an "inward" mindset that dehumanizes others and puts unrealistic expectations on themselves. This is why many responders intuitively connect with Arbinger tools and philosophy. Responders, their families, and agencies immediately see the benefit of learning new ways to communicate and think about problems. It gives them hope and motivation when the future includes fewer walls, isolation, anger, and scorekeeping in their relationships.

Developing an "outward" mind is connected to the third concept of resilience. As mentioned before, when we perceive that others are a constant threat to us and our happiness or that they have some kind of control over our emotions, we are constantly on guard. Maintaining that kind of stance wears on our bodies and minds and increases the chances of negative consequences to our physical and mental health. We all too frequently see disturbing statistics about responder suicide rates, injuries, and decisions that are often connected to job-related stress or injuries. Shifting mindset doesn't just improve work performance, personal satisfaction, teamwork, relationships, and heal families; it can increase resilience, lower dependence on self-medication, and potentially save lives.

Increasing resilience is also about changing our relationship with stress. We teach clients that stress is normal. Thus, instead of running and blaming others for the stress to make it go away, we can pay attention to it, acknowledge it, and use awareness to become more efficient flowing with it and use it to our benefit.

Pearson explains that popular culture is programming people to believe they cannot change their relationship to stress.

Tremendous emotional and physical pressure will crack anyone. Responders and others are conditioned to think that the best way to protect their families and friends from seeing them crack under the pressure is to bottle up emotion, hide the side effects, and double down on work and "toughness." With these beliefs in play, it makes sense that more police officers get divorced than the national average. It also sheds light as to why families don't personally know or understand the emotional walls and other coping mechanisms being applied by their responders in their efforts to keep going, but only see that they are falling apart in front of their eyes.

Chateau Recovery tries to help responders and other clients with four forms of stress/trauma that significantly impact life. Developmental stress, also known as toxic stress, is connected to situations or conditions, often related to neglect or abuse, that someone may have endured during their childhood. Those experiences often impact how a child grows, views themselves, and interacts with the world around them. The Chateau uses specialized assessment tools to help target developmental events that need to be addressed in treatment. Vicarious trauma is a common challenge for responders or anyone who is frequently exposed to violence or victims of trauma. As mentioned earlier, constant exposure to intense and dehumanizing situations and suffering alters mindset and resilience in profoundly negative ways. Generational or intergenerational stress and trauma is related to thinking and behavioral patterns that are perpetuated within family systems, which can create powerful and lasting negative impacts. The last category of stress is the more popularly known stressors that are unfortunate and impersonal events occurring from challenges, accidents, or daily expectations. These negatively impact individuals and families in different ways but are impersonal in nature. Any of these kinds of stressors can contribute to post-traumatic stress disorder or post-traumatic stress injuries and need to be addressed by professionals. Regardless of which constellation of stressors clients experience prior to coming to the Chateau, our job is to help them slow down, find new tools to help them get grounded, start confronting issues and beliefs, and help them develop some new insights and awareness. All clients successfully completing the program have an individually created plan for continuing to build and nurture a mindset and skill set that is flexible and resilient as they are faced with challenges in their journey beyond the Chateau.

Most of the clients come into the program having a specific idea of a specific behavior or problem that they believe is "the problem." Days later, after completing assessments and interviews that explore personality traits, trauma, values, and other aspects of the program, they usually have a perspective shift and recognize that their work is more important and complicated than they expected. Many responders realize, often for the first time, that there are many issues in their life that needed to be addressed, but didn't understand their urgency, impact, or where to start. That same sentiment is also true when it comes to returning home. After a transformative experience in treatment, they often need direction and support in applying new ideas to home and work. Many clients are unaware of how comprehensive their home- and work-life plans needs to be in order for life to get better. To this end, as mentioned above, the Chateau guides each client through the process of creating their individual *Self-Leadership Plan* that encapsulates the concepts, tools, values, and commitments they connected within the program. This plan lays out strengths and weaknesses and new self-care habits they commit to keeping in each dimension of their life. It also highlights high-risk situations and regression signs that are likely in the near future at home and work. Since they are the architects of this plan and they are the ones who need to recruit and assign responsibilities to those within their system, each responder is asked to explain their plan to family members, their ongoing mental health provider, and their home agency peer support person. Within that process, they also give their support team permission to get involved if regressions signs appear, and plan on regular check-ins to stay on track. This way, the individual leaving treatment is the one deciding how much personal information is shared and how far the support goes into work situations. The track record of this system is strong, and responders and agencies that have used this plan report feeling empowered and supported in this challenging transition time.

Our goal for the client is to have a deeper and more accurate outlook on who they are as a person and who they want to be by the time they leave the program. We focus on what makes them unique, what kind of values they have, and what they can accomplish in each dimension of their life. We educate them on healthy ways to deal with stress when it arises, and we provide an environment that allows mistakes and learning from experience. We help them become more creative in their ability to find health and resilience. We help them initiate self-care and introduce proper nutrition, mindfulness, mediation, and yoga. We explain the importance of sleep and exercise. We help them grow and practice a new mindset and sense of ownership of their lives. We teach and help them develop skills to communicate with their family and friends in a healthier manner. Through realistic expectations, patience, and a positive mindset, our clients can see solutions to their efforts instead of old excuses, blame, or barriers. Our clients are taught to anticipate struggles instead of pretending that they will not encounter them anymore if they go to treatment. We help them create a plan of action for when those anticipated struggles arise again in their lives. We help them have a healthy relationship with stress. Within all the above, clients begin to have a more compassionate view of themselves. Thus, when they do encounter struggles in life, they have tools that will aid them in being more flexible in their ability to deal with them.

Thayer Crouse, Director of Development and Outreach for the Chateau Recovery Treatment Center, elaborates on some of these details.

Traditionally, the way Chateau Recovery receives calls for assistance from first responders themselves or from their own police agency. The calls range from small to large police departments across the country. Chateau Recovery also receives calls from peer support teams and from smaller law enforcement agencies that do not have the necessary mental health resources available.

We receive a phone call from an individual in emotional crisis when the first responder realizes they cannot get better on their own. That officer needs a treatment center to get the mental and emotional support they need. Ninety-nine percent of police officers, firefighters, and first responders are in complete crisis when they call our facility. Most often, they are on the verge of losing their job, their marriage, or everything they have worked so hard for most of their life. These first responders are not only being proactive, but they are seeking our help by saying, "Hey, I'm struggling, I need help now!" Emotionally troubled first responders are ready to come to our facility and get the help and treatment they need.

We usually take a quick preliminary assessment over the phone, immediately taking care of any insurance issues and concerns they may have. We arrange for that first responder to get to our facility as quickly and as safely as they can, usually in a matter of hours. First responders often fear their agency will find out they are seeking mental health treatment. Everything, including treatment, is absolutely confidential for all who attend Chateau Recovery.

When police officers or firefighters arrive, they are given an initial assessment that includes basic questions primarily dealing with the mental health and trauma issues they might have experienced. We also discuss any reoccurring anxiety and depression. An abundance of first responders who seek treatment show signs of PTSD. Officers who come in for our substance-abuse program will normally be for alcohol-related issues. There have been a few instances of opiate substance-abuse cases related to addiction from injury-related problems. We are finding that most of the officers who come to our facility are in the ninth or tenth year of service. They are having a difficult time on the job and at home.

Lately, not many young men or women are interested in becoming police officers. Many law enforcement agencies are hiring former military veterans. The military veterans who are now in law enforcement come with a lot more baggage from the war. We are now finding the average years of service for police officers who have military experience are often seeking therapy with only three, four, or five years on the job. At Chateau, we have progressive ideas and concepts for these officers with previous military experience. We want these officers to get healthy with all that they have gone through. Frankly, it is a huge letdown because many of the officers who were in the military are not taken care of appropriately in our society.

Most officers understand the stigma of not coming forward for help, therapy, or treatment for emotional support. It is pretty well documented across the board. I want people to know about the solutions that are out there. That does not necessarily mean inpatient treatment services. Unfortunately, for most people in crisis, in-house recovery is necessary. Chateau offers individual therapy and a program called Stepstone Connect. This program is an intensive outpatient treatment, and they also provide responder assistance programs, similar to an employee assistance program (EAP). The Stepstone Connect program is all through video conferencing. Officers, firefighters, and first responders alike can get help from the privacy of their own home. If a police officer on duty feels they need a remedial session, they can take a break and access the session privately on the phone in their squad car. We are trying to take the innovative solutions to them and to make it as easy as possible for them to feel safe asking for help.

Crouse believes in the six distinct dimensions of resiliency that Chateau has to offer its clients. With trauma being at the center of everyone's life, these six dimensions are connected and intertwined with each other.

We believe trauma spurs most things, whether it is alcohol, drug addiction, depression, or PTSD. When a first responder comes to our facility, our initial assessment give us a good idea where they are mentally and emotionally on our wellness scale.

The first dimension sets the tone early in regards to the officer's mental and emotional mindset. It is important to understand the issues that may have traumatized the officer. The troubled officer who is in crisis most often has been plagued with many problematic issues, for quite some time, most often even before their law enforcement career. Did the officer seek help on their own, or were they remanded by their department to get help for their emotional troubles? An important part of the first dimension is the importance of self-acceptance, motivation, and psychological flexibility. One important factor in the treatment and rehabilitation of most first responders is to recognize and identify their goals, skills, and motivators for seeking help. This will assist the psychologists and counselors to help these officers overcome any personal challenges they were experiencing. The purpose of emotional wellness is to live a long and healthy life with the ability to handle day-to-day stress and reoccurring depression.

First responders who come to the facility are concerned with their nutrition and physical activity, so the second-dimension enables them to incorporate physical activity, diet, and nutrition in their routine to get healthy. One of the first questions they ask is, "Do we get to go to a gym?" The answer is yes, they do, six to seven days a week.

— CHAPTER 9 —

PEER SUPPORT AND OTHER

EMPLOYEE ASSISTANCE OPTIONS

They say a person needs just three things to be truly happy in this world.
Someone to love, something to do, and something to hope for.
Tom Bodett

POLICE OFFICERS HAVE one thing in common: they do not trust many people. Officers face numerous conflicts on a day-to-day basis, which often causes their demeanor to become hardened slowly over time. Who better to assist and understand a police officer than one of their peers? An officer is more likely to speak with a fellow officer than with a psychologist or trained professional, often because they do not want to appear weak or chance losing their job.

In the early stages of peer support, police officers were reluctant to tell anyone about the tragedies, crime scenes, and death they witnessed and experienced. As a peer support team member and team leader, I have spoken with many police officers who were struggling with many emotional issues. These officers felt comfortable confiding in me, and they trusted me because they knew their problems would be held in confidence.

Peer support officers have been extensively trained to assist police officers and their immediate families in a crisis situation. Peer support officers are trained to never judge their fellow officers and are there to show support as they try to understand the negative mindset of the troubled officer. A peer support team member will never write anything down and can reassure the officer in crisis by always adhering to a strict code of confidence.

Peer support addresses depression, anxiety, marital and financial problems, drinking and alcoholism, sleep-related issues, and all other stresses related to the job. If the peer support team member feels the officer needs more emotional assistance than they can provide, they can always turn to one of the professional in-house psychologists or therapists in the Employee Assistance Program (EAP) or an on-call police chaplain or counselor.

Peer support team members help the troubled officers address and cope with the issue at hand by being active listeners. It is important for all peer support team members to ensure they follow up their initial visit with a phone call or a recommendation of available options that the troubled officer can benefit from.

Benefits of Peer Support Systems

- Police will most likely confide in other police officers.
- No notes and complete confidentiality.
- Immediate on scene emotional awareness.
- Active listening, communication is imperative.
- Availability can be 24/7, 365 days a year.

Dr. Jack Digliani explains.

Police officers have supported one another since the inception of police forces. In the early years when police officers experienced emotional difficulties or troubling stressors, whether or not work-related, they could always rely on the traditional booze and buddies (B and B) for solace. The results produced by the B and B method of stress management were sometimes less than desirable. Although booze and buddies still exist today, police officers now have several alternatives for assistance when dealing with stress-related difficulties. In many contemporary police agencies, these alternatives include the option of working with members of the department's peer support team. Police peer support teams have proven their worth and have demonstrated their effectiveness for many years. They have established their place in the police mentality and have become an integral part of many law enforcement agencies.

Peer support teams occupy a support niche that cannot be readily filled by either an EAP, health plan provisions, or a police psychologist. If an agency wants to do the best it can to support its officers, a peer support team is necessary. Incidentally, a peer support team is one of the most valued resources for a police agency staff psychologist—many staff psychologist counseling and preemptive intervention programs are designed to incorporate the efficacy of peer support.

Barbara Arkwright, Special Agent in Charge with the Department of Motor Vehicles in Richmond, Virginia, says,

> Peer support professionals are not hindered by employment laws or department human resources policies, like management can be. They are the bridge between the officer who is experiencing trauma or just the everyday stress of life and a professional referral for assistance. A good peer support professional not only understands their role but also their limitations. They are not "fixers." They are trained to actively listen without judgment and maintain confidentiality. When necessary, they assist with making referrals to doctors, financial advisors, chaplains, and police psychologists who understand and can relate to an officer in crisis.

I have had many great mentors throughout my career; some provided peer support to me and may have never even known it. One is famous for his quote, "When the public needs help, they call the police. When the police need help, who do they call? Each other!" It is true, it is easier for police officers to open up to someone they feel a bond with, someone they can relate to. Police officers, in some ways, are no different from anyone else when it comes to life stressors. An officer who is suffering from an addiction or who suffers with a loved one who has an addiction, an officer who is grieving the loss of a loved one or is comforting a family member because they are the strong one, an officer who is depressed and maybe contemplating suicide or living with someone with depression who may have suicidal tendencies. Suffering from anxiety due to life challenges is not unique. However, police officers seem to be distinctive in a way that they self-identify based on their profession.

Another mentor shared a poignant observation he would hear at parties and gatherings. The conversation would go like this: "What is your occupation?" Most people would answer, "I work for the police." Officers normally would respond proudly, "I am a police officer." His observation was, "We are the job." Everyone in our neighborhood knows who we are. We are always in the public eye whether we are on duty or not. That is a tremendous burden to carry on a daily basis. The same mentor shared with me his philosophy of being a police officer was akin to balancing oneself on a three-legged stool. The first leg is the officer, the second is "the officer's family/friends/support mechanism, and the third is the job. His analogy was that a police officer is so intertwined with their job as part of their self-identity and their life that if one leg were to be removed, the stool would collapse and the officer would be at a tipping point. Each person reacts to stress in their own way; what is traumatic for one person may not be for another. Exposure to trauma and everyday stressors cannot be eliminated, but they can be managed. Some people are more resilient than others due to previous trauma they have dealt with and overcome and are stronger for those experiences.

Lieutenant Frank Scarpa, Richmond (Virginia) Police Department, shares how his department addresses officers seeking emotional help.

Officers seeking emotional help has gotten better, probably in the last three years or so. We have implemented the *Road to Resilience Program* (R2R). This program deals with trauma that police officers encounter, including the day-to-day exposure to calls for service dealing with violence, harassment from the public, scrutiny, bad management, and in some cases a difficult home life. For the most part, the mindset in the Richmond Police Department is similar to that in the Chicago Police Department, that it is not macho or manly to seek help. If a police officer has experienced something tragic, they most likely will keep it to themselves and not talk about it, especially if it is affecting them emotionally. We need to change that; we need to make sure that officers are getting the support and help they need. They need to be able to come out from their dark place and say, *"I NEED HELP!"* without worrying about backlash from the department, or whispering behind officers' backs about being mentally weak.

Emotional wellness is getting better with the newer, younger officers being hired. They feel more comfortable talking about their feelings. Over the years, whether I was an officer or supervisor, I would make recommendations to an officer who seemed distraught to seek out a counselor or mental health professional. But most officers have that same mindset and would say, "I'm fine, I'm fine, I'll figure it out, I'll go to a bar drinking and I will feel better on Monday." This is exactly the opposite of what we want officers to do, to deal with their emotions by pouring alcohol all over it.

Chris Scallon, retired sergeant with the Norfolk (Virginia) Police Department, says,

> I received ten thousand dollars to start up a peer support program. Someone told me that establishing a peer support unit was like flying a plane while building it because issues exist during implementation.
>
> I soon realized that everything becomes compartmentalized; I have yet to run into an officer who is struggling with one problem. No one has just one issue. There may be a guy or girl who is struggling with a specific incident. These problems just don't start on the job, they occur when that person is growing up. Life is life, and people need to assign blame. I grew up in Brooklyn in the 1980s with a violent culture, and gun shots rang out often. It is pretty much what Chicago is like today. Everything has an impact, family, life, everything.

Kurt Gawrisch, a certified Crisis Intervention Team (CIT) state instructor and coordinator, says,

> If a department has a peer support program, it may be one of the best kept secrets. Sometimes peer support is a secret due to lack of awareness, fear of stigma, or limited understanding on access, which leads to underutilization. Officers are hesitant asking for help because of the fear of the unknowns, wondering what's going to happen. When promoting the program, it's important to explain the step-by-step process so officers know what they are walking into. When officers use peer support, they should discover 24-hour support, a judgment-free setting, and individuals who understand the law enforcement work environment. Peer support complements an employee assistance program but does not replace it.

Father Dan Brandt, director of the Chicago Police Chaplain's Unit, suggests another support option.

> We are taking proactive measures to help our officers deal with issues they are facing by offering prayer services for every different

religious denomination almost every day of the week. We want to feed the soul through prayer. We offer marriage retreats, marriage seminars, and cancer survivor workshops, as well as suicide awareness seminars. I have been involved in a day-long officer-involved shooting class for the past ten years. The first half of the class we speak about post-traumatic stress, the law and being sued, the spiritual side of ending a life, and the difference between the killing of a person and murder of a person. We emphasize they did not shoot to kill but shot to live. We bring in officers who were involved in previous police shootings to hear their stories and how they have coped with the stress and trauma afterward. Many of the officers in the class have the opportunity to share what transpired with everyone attending. This class is helpful and therapeutic because their feedback gives us examples of what is needed and helpful for future officers involved in shootings. The second half of the program is held in the range for enhanced tactical training. The Chicago Police Department supports and encourages any officer involved in a police-related shooting to attend this important program.

Jack A. Digliani, PhD, EdD, is an advocate for a proactive annual check-in (PAC).

> PAC provides police officers and other agency employees with a confidential setting within which to share information about current life circumstances. It is a proactive program designed to offer a positive exchange of thoughts, ideas, and information. The six elements of the PAC are as follows.
>
> 1. Annual visit with the staff psychologist, a member of the peer support team, department chaplain, private counselor, or other support resource,
> 2. Confidential meeting that does not initiate any record,
> 3. No evaluation—It's a *check-in*, not a *checkup*,

4. There does not need to be a problem,

5. It's a discussion of what's happening in the officer's life, and

6. Participation is voluntary and encouraged. (Note: although participation in the PAC program was designed to be entirely voluntary, some police agencies are experimenting with making annual support contacts mandatory. Other agencies are providing incentives for voluntary participation, such as rewarding participants with vacation time.)

– CHAPTER 10 –

BECOMING HEATHIER IN EVERY WAY

Be aware of what others are doing, applaud their efforts,
acknowledge their successes, and encourage them in their
pursuits. When we all help one another, everybody wins.
Jim Stovall

LIFE IS TOO SHORT to be unhappy. To have a happy and fulfilling life is not about the amount of money officers take home or the promotions they attain, but it is about their positive disposition, which matters most. Every officer needs purpose in their life, and it is important for them to aspire to make a positive difference in the world in which they live. Actor Denzel Washington once said, "Dreams without goals are just dreams."

POLICE WELLNESS

In my opinion, police wellness must first deal with an officer's disposition and outlook on life. Earlier in the book I mentioned how police officers may start out happy, but later in their careers it becomes obvious that their disposition have changed. How ironic that almost every class in every police academy focuses on police tactics and survival on the streets, but few, if any, classes focus on the police officer's well-being or their state of mind from what they may encounter in their career.

Police wellness starts with attaining a better disposition. We must give officers the opportunity to better themselves from the destructive nature of the job. I have noticed throughout my career how the outlook on law enforcement has changed for many of my fellow officers. Officers seem more critical and bitter about the career they have chosen. Many are disheartened and dissatisfied going to work. Many officers who have been in law enforcement for quite some time have gradually lost their enthusiasm for the job, and, it seems, for life itself. In my opinion, quite a few officers with twenty-five or more years of service have become opinionated, belligerent, and downright mean. It's no wonder that many of the younger officers can't wait until these older, grouchy cops retire.

THE POWER OF OPTIMISM

In a TEDx talk titled "The Power of Optimism,"[9] Bert Jacobs presents what I believe is a great introduction into police wellness. Bert speaks about the importance of optimism and how a person can create their own happiness and overcome obstacles just by being optimistic. He shared a few stories about when he was a youngster growing up. He says his mom was truly optimistic and positive when it came to raising her children. His mom gave Bert and his siblings the opportunity to explore and discover their vivid imaginations. He explained that his mom would ask everyone seated at the dinner table to "Tell me something good that happened today." He said those seven simple words changed the energy in their home.

Bert pointed out that the media almost always points out what is wrong in the world, yet rarely speaks about what is right. He mentioned that we have a choice: we can focus on the negative and what is wrong with our lives, or we can focus on the positive and see what is right with them. That statement made me think how police officers gradually change overtime because of what they deal with throughout their career.

I believe many police officers get into a negative routine that affects everyone they come into contact with. My dad had a philosophy similar to Bert Jacobs's. I remember my dad telling me a valuable story a few days before I was about to attend high school. He told me that when I wake up in the morning that I

---

[9] https://www.youtube.com/watch?v=yYGNWIT4eqA

could either be happy or sad. "It's your choice," he said. "You have the ability to choose to start your day being either happy or sad, positive or negative." Everyone gravitates to a happy and friendly person, he explained. My dad was a positive person in my life. From that day forward, I chose to be happy no matter what the day brought me, even though there were days that I experienced sadness and heartache. When those days occurred, I always remembered my dad and our positive conversation. It always helped in many stressful situations.

In my opinion, Bert Jacobs's words are truly inspirational. He points out that an optimistic person understands opportunity and learns to overcome obstacles and adversity. He explains that an optimistic person is more open-minded and innovative, and they are not afraid to experiment and explore the world. He gives a compelling example of an eleven-year-old girl who was inflicted with bone cancer that ravaged her young body. Her prognosis was not good, and doctors gave her less than a year to live. She said that before she got sick, she took her life for granted. This young girl was often seen wearing a cap because of her hair loss from the chemotherapy injected into her body. Her baseball cap read; Life Is Good. This saying was a reminder to her to stay positive and happy. It was her optimism for life that accessed her courage. She beat the cancer and is a happy and cheerful teenager today.

Vickie Poklop, a police counselor with the Des Plaines, (Illinois) Police Department, says,

> Police wellness is a great big category, and police officers are sometimes uncomfortable with some of the things that are becoming more mainstream these days, like meditation, yoga, and being mindful. These are really fantastic coping skills, if officers are willing to just give them a try. Unwind, sit down, meditate, or relax to a quiet inner world. The world out there is hectic and so crazy, and officers are in that environment all day long.

Eric Ramirez-Thompson, PhD, agrees.

> I would like to see more officers learn about the mind and body connection in their training in the police academy. The research

shows that police officers still see themselves as enforcers and pro-tectors with a warrior-type mentality. New and seasoned officers who overlook the importance of physical and spiritual well-being are at risk of never achieving the highest levels of personal and professional success. The ever-changing nature of law enforce-ment requires that academy training include an emphasis on healthy living.

Dara N. Rampersad, PhD, LPC, NCC, says,

Wellness encompasses a sense of belonging, purpose, high self-efficacy, feeling like you're making a difference, and hav-ing the support of your administration and coworkers, etc. A police officer's mental wellness can be affected if they feel they are failing at their job on a weekly or monthly basis because officers do not have the support to do their job as well as they think they should.

Speaking across the board, about 95% of first responder personalities are Type A. They are high-achieving individuals with a strong desire to win. They want to be on the forefront of trying to solve problems quickly. They want to have the resources to take care of problems fast, be successful, and put a patch or Band-Aid on the problem and move to the next problem. First responders are crisis driven individuals; they generally do not want to be bogged down by a call or crime scene that will occupy them for hours. For the most part, patrol officers want to know that they have the support to get the job done quickly, efficiently, and good enough to move on to the next call.

I think an officer's wellness is severely affected because their job is impacted by their environment and by feeling unsupported in trying to make a difference in what they are doing. Everyone in the world, whether they are a first responder or not, needs to have a sense of purpose, needs to know their purpose is being achieved through their meaningful actions.

Reverend Timothy F. Perry, President of 10-41, Incorporated, created the 10-41 Physical, Intellectual, Emotional, and Spiritual (PIES) Wellness Approach. He believes there are four types of answers to any problems:

Physical: Maintain physical activity to generate the chemicals like dopamine to impact your mind and body.

Intellectual: Engage in collecting information and validate it with a mental health practitioner or chaplain.

Emotional: We can always connect with a chaplain or counselor.

Spiritual: Those that are faith-based may opt to use spiritual leaders from a church, synagogue, temple, etc. Sometimes spiritual emotions can be drawn from being in an environment that soothes the heart, mind, and soul. These are places like a mountain top or the seashore.

Chris Taliaferro, 29th Ward Alderman and former Chicago Police officer, says,

> One of my biggest concerns with the nature of the job is the impact of wellness on our police officers. I have served twenty-one years as a police officer, and I understand the position a lot of officers have been put in and the issues that they deal with at work and at home. The impact of an officer's well-being is a major concern right now. I am impressed by the Los Angeles Police Department and the way that they have handled mental wellness issues and concerns in their department. They have gone almost two years without a police suicide. They are doing something right. All police departments across the country should emulate their proactive and positive system of addressing police mental health.
>
> The Los Angeles Police Department's behavioral health system is quite different than what we have in Chicago. Los Angeles uses highly trained and licensed police psychologists. These police psychologists spend a lot of time and effort in getting to know and build relationships with their officers. When this occurs, officers are more likely to open up to them when an issue arises.

It is similar to a friendship-type plan where they become more approachable when an officer is in need of psychological or emotional help. That philosophy makes a huge difference, and it has produced positive results. Los Angeles is not looking to strip an officer of their police powers if they seek assistance for any emotional problems that an officer may be experiencing.

We have to do what Los Angeles Police Department has been able to accomplish. Their behavioral science section does not relieve an officer of their police responsibilities but instead works to ensure the officer is mentally safe from harm and still treated for their emotional issues at the same time. It is not only a call to our current model, but a call to the State of Illinois to give officers the opportunity to address mental health concerns without being placed in jeopardy of losing the FOID card, and essentially their job. This is perhaps one of the leading reasons many officers refuse to even talk to anyone about issues that may be bothering them.

EMOTIONAL RESILIENCE

As Vickie Poklop explains,

Emotional resilience is something that all people can learn. There is a balance between being emotionally resilient and releasing negative emotions. If we hang onto the hurtful words or experiences we have had, then at some point they will control us. Working through those experiences and emotions with a trusted mental health professional allows us to release the pain of the past and to forge a future without the weight of past turmoil. Nobody gets through life unscarred, and it is not a badge of honor to carry emotional pain around with us for our entire lives. Imagine the freedom that comes from letting go of past hurts.

HOLISTIC HEALING

Rosa Cortez, owner of Naperville Healing Center, is an Eastern medicine practitioner and a tenth-generation Mayan healer who believes in a whole-body approach to holistic healing. She believes the whole-body approach to healing helps police officers who are already going through stress, PTSD, and adrenal and chronic fatigue. Rosa is also a certified yoga instructor, reflexologist, Reiki Energy Master Teacher who listens to a person's body and helps align it back to homeostasis.

I incorporate different holistic treatment modalities. Yoga unites a person's mind and body. Reflexology helps align a person's organs and meridians by clearing the channels that correspond to a specific organ. Reiki energy healing and the Mayan healing targets the energy centers of the body and aligns and clears the channels energetically. The body is always talking, revealing what is wrong. My approach has helped many police officers reduce their adrenal fatigue because they are constantly in a fight or flight mode. They experience an enormous amount of stress because of their job. They almost never relax, and I get them to relax and heal their underlying issues with every session.

Everyone always takes from a police officer, and police officers rarely take for themselves. How many police officers go to a holistic healer, take a yoga class, practice meditation, see an acupuncturist, or even get a massage to work on their stress and deal with their underlying trauma? I'm sure not many. Self-love is vital for an officer's health.

A person's diet is very important, but to be on the right diet is essential. Many people get on the wrong diet because they do not listen to their bodies and what their bodies are lacking. Most officers suffer from weight problems after a couple of years on the job. A majority of officers overeat because of stress and anxiety from doing their job. Excess weight represents trauma, and a person holding onto trauma often gains weight and becomes obese.

A person who overeats is lacking something. Sometimes they don't eat at all or have only one meal a day if that. Yet they continue to gain weight. They feel bloated, sluggish, and start having insecurity issues due to the weight gain. Weight gain is a security response, a sign of adrenal fatigue.

Disease corelates to an emotion as the root cause, and healing that emotion allows the body to heal. Police officers need to take time for themselves, love themselves, and allow their bodies to heal.

Exercise

I am amazed to see how many overweight cops are working in law enforcement. I came to realize that I was putting on quite a few pounds and joining that group. Was it the stress of the job, poor eating habits, or not working out or exercising like I should have been? Many police officers probably will not like my next suggestion. My suggestion for a healthier and happier police department is to make it mandatory for all officers to stay in shape. They should have to pass a fitness test once a year, like the Illinois State Police do, to keep their job. This is the incentive for all officers to work harder, eat better, and stay healthier. They would most likely have a better lifestyle because of it.

When I completed my twenty-five weeks in the Chicago Police Academy, I was forty years old and in the best shape of my life. I was 6 ft. tall, 175 lbs., with a thirty-four-inch waist and solid. I was surprised to find out that after I graduated from the police academy that I was not obligated to participate in any more annual physical fitness exams. It wasn't mandatory but voluntary for a fitness award and $200. I only tried for and received one fitness award in my entire twenty-two-year career. Shame on me as I look back on what I should have done.

The Illinois State Police Troopers have an annual exam not only for weight but also for physical fitness that is required for future employment. I believe that every police department should have the same mandatory policy. I have to admit that I started gaining weight after I left the Academy. There was no excuse—it was easy to blame a thirty-minute lunch/dinner enjoying fast food and unhealthy eating. I made excuses for not working out and keeping in shape. I would say that I had court, school, working overtime, and side jobs. I was also ashamed of seeing some of my fellow officers at roll call, on the street, or on TV with their stomachs hanging out past their bulletproof vests. I soon realized that I was becoming that officer and should lose weight.

John M. Violanti, PhD, agrees that lack of exercise is a problem.

The life expectancy of police officers is a major indication that that there are health problems in law enforcement, and we need to do something about that. When we did our first police life expectancy study, we found that police officers were dying at a much earlier age than the general population. Even around middle age, fifty to sixty years of age, officers were dying. Another study we did recently found that because of on-duty exposures like having to chase people or sudden stress, officers were having heart attacks. A study we did over twenty-one years found that the average age of a heart attack while on duty or related to duty was around forty-seven years of age. Something is wrong here, and what can we do? How are we going to convince a police officer to stay healthy? When we talk to police officers they will say, "Yeah, yeah, yeah, I know that I have to eat more salads, I've got to exercise, and I've got to sleep better."

Many officers get the attitude of "Well, I know this stuff that is necessary to stay healthy, but I don't do it." The trick is to change negative attitudes into positive behavior. A lot of this can start with the organization; we are way behind compared to industry putting up wellness programs. We are starting to do it now. I have seen more and more wellness programs coming out recently. This is essential, and important when the officer first comes into the job at the academy level. To get the attitude and the behavior set at that point have it carried on through the twenty to twenty-five years that the officer may spend in law enforcement is imperative. Wellness programs are good, they teach people what to do and how to do it. That is essential for officers right now.

Coach Sok (Bruce Sokolove), agrees.

> I spend most of the year in a classroom with police officers who averaged eight to ten years on the job. I have never seen a more at-risk law enforcement population as much as I am looking at in the last ten years of American policing. These guys are not healthy. Their risk of cardiovascular disease is over the top, with many who are obese and have, or on a rapid path toward, type 2 diabetes. Their lifestyle, including poor eating habits, is not conducive to tactical fitness in any way. If these guys would just understand how much they could knock down their cortisol (a primary stress hormone) levels with a regimen of daily exercise. It is not necessary to train like an Olympian, but only forty minutes of brisk walking, some lightweight training, or any type of physical exercise would be ideal. Look at the number of cops we lose every year because of coronary heart disease. It is sad and maddening.

There is evidence suggesting that male police officers are at a higher risk of developing coronary disease than males in the general population.[10] In an article published in CopsAlive.com, Jonathon Sheinberg, MD, a board-certified cardiologist and lieutenant of the Lakeway, Texas, Police Department, writes, "Heart attacks are always in the top two or three categories of police line of duty deaths."[11]

In a personal conversation, Dr. Sheinberg told me,

> Here is the problem: there is a handful of limited data about the actual number of heart attacks that police officer incur in law enforcement. In law enforcement, heart attacks are the number

---

[10]   Sparrow, D. (1983); Veterans Administration Outpatient Clinic, Boston Ma. Study: Coronary heart disease in police officers participating in Normative Aging Study, Am J Epidemiol 1983; 1983: 508-13.

[11]   Sheinberg, Jonathan MD. FACC,(2015) Heart Disease and the Law Enforcement Officer,CopsAlive.com, August 31, 2015 Plan Your Health.

one cause of death among police officers. It is difficult to track because most death are categorized as line of duty deaths. When someone mentions a heart attack, most people think of the cause as a blocked artery. When someone has a heart attack, plaque forms on the walls of arteries. The wall of the artery gets inflamed and that plague erupts and bursts. A clot then forms, and that clot blocks the blood flow. That is what a heart attack is.[12]

Dr. Sheinberg believes there is something about our law enforcement that drives this process to accelerate to a higher level.

Police officers for the most part have a sedentary job. Their stress pattern on patrol is 98% boredom punctuated by 2% terror. They may be involved in a situation that will take them from 0 to 100 miles an hour in a short time. Their blood pressure elevates and their stress response causes a physiological change that causes the plaque in the arteries to rupture. Because of this, we are seeing heart attacks in younger police officers more frequently.

The life expectancy of police officers is twenty-two years less than the general population. The average age for a heart attack for police officers is forty-six years old, compared to the middle-to-late sixties for the general population of the United States. Dr. John Violanti mentions in his research on police mortality that a civilian who is between the ages of fifty-five and fifty-nine has a 1.6% of dying from a heart attack. If you are a cop, it is at 56%. We see a thirty-seven-fold increase in death at that age. I found myself perfectly positioned to study this because I am a doctor as well as a police officer. What I started doing was looking at early markers of heart disease in law enforcement now, and not waiting to collect data after the officer died. We are trying to collect data early, and I am finding the disproportionate influence of early heart disease in the police

---

[12] Jonathon Sheinberg, MD, in a personal conversation on October 17, 2020.

population. Heart attacks are increasing earlier and more often in a police officer's career than ever before.

Coach Sok doesn't think heart disease should be inevitable.

Life collides, excuses are made. "I don't have time, I'm busy." The physical training and exercise they did at the police academy are no longer mandated. So a lot of cops do not work out or exercise as they did preparing for certification. An unfit cop is not a safe cop. I am talking across the board to include mental health as well as physical health. It is a lot easier to pack on the pounds than to take it off and keep it off. I recently spoke with Dr. Kevin Gilmartin and asked him if he could wave a magic wand over the soon-to-be-minted street cops, what would he prescribe for them? He said, "Two things: number one, every cop would be assigned to a vetted police psychologist for regular mental health check-ins, and number two, each officer would be assigned a fitness-and nutrition-coordinator throughout their career." I concur that Dr. Gilmartin's philosophy would be beneficial. I am convinced there would have fewer injuries, on-duty incidents, and fewer disability retirements. This initiative would pay for itself.

We need to ensure that our officers get back into shape and stay in shape. It would have to involve physical fitness while the officers are on duty. That could be a sticking point; I have been around the United States teaching and have visited many police facilities with state-of-the-art training equipment, and there is hardly anyone using it. It is not realistic for an officer to try to work out in a gym or at the station during their lunch because of time constraints and calls the dispatcher is holding for them upon their return.

Maybe a solution is to take the cost benefit analysis of allowing our police personnel to work out before shift (compensated). Get their endorphins popping. Get a good workout, hit the shower, put on the uniform, then roll call and hit the street. That might be the best part of their shift, quite frankly, because their day may go downhill after that.

There is a lot of empirical research on fitness that could be used as reasonable age/gender-adjusted, job-related standards. Imagine the number of injuries on duty departments are seeing because of the lack of physical fitness. And the rise in the number of worker compensation claims, in-service training injuries, particularly during defensive tactics. Just look at the personnel we lose annually due to cardiac events during training. Hope and wishing are not a plan for success. Police officers (as well as retired officers) need to have a sensible plan and support system to get back into shape and stay in shape.

Dr. Eric Ramirez-Thompson believes exercise is an effective alternative to prescribed and self-administered medications like alcohol.

Any form of exercise removes a person from behaviors and activities associated with trauma. Exercise can recalibrate the release of neurotransmitters that become abundant as a result of trauma. With this being said, yoga can be a helpful coping strategy for officers, where they can center themselves and literally take time to relax.

The healing process takes time and does not happen overnight; the brain has to rewire itself in order to deal with stress. They must learn various ways to remove themselves from conditions that trigger an emotional response and counteract autonomic cognitive reactions that affect thoughts, feelings, and behavior. Such work requires commitment, and they must spend a lot of time working on coping strategies that hold the potential to reorganize communication pathways in the brain. Exercise not only benefits us physiologically, but there are also behavioral therapy benefits. In the research that I did years ago that involved the benefits of exercise, I discovered that exercising activates natural neurochemicals such as serotonin. The body needs physical activity and exercise to be able to release these neurochemicals to needed levels.

Healthy Eating

Nutrition was never mentioned or discussed in the police academy. The importance of eating healthy and maintaining a healthy lifestyle should be part of the police curriculum. Officers are more likely to be in a higher risk level for heart attack, stroke, and type 2 diabetes because of the pitfalls associated with a poor diet and the stress of the job.

Nutrition expert Dr. Justin Gruby explains:

> Police officers have a unique occupation because of their schedule, which can often lead to biochemical, physical, and mental stress. When an officer experiences burnout or a loss of energy, or is not sleeping well, it is possible the adrenal glands may not be functioning properly. The adrenal glands secrete many hormones, and one of them is called cortisol, which is the stress hormone. We need cortisol to live and to be able to respond to normal stimuli in our environment. However, when a person has too much stress, testing will often show an elevated cortisol level, which increases a person's ability to feel pain, increase their blood pressure and blood sugar levels, and can create a major health crisis. I regularly order testing that will measure an officer's cortisol level to better determine the function of the adrenal glands.

> Eating healthy can be a challenge for many officers. The problem most officers have is with what they eat and when they eat. Their routine often includes checking in the station, have something sugary as they grab a cup of coffee to start their day. For lunch or dinner, they often stop at fast-food places because of time constraints. They have to really be dedicated and strict to stay away from the bad stuff. Officers need to change their routines because they often don't get the basic nutritional requirements from day to day to keep inflammation at bay. I can almost

guarantee you that you are not going to find cut up carrots or celery on the dash of a squad car.

The old saying, "You are what you eat" is true. Another issue that is affecting our health and nutrition is the food quality. One of my patients said he likes buying large bags of tilapia and other frozen fish. The issue arises when the fish are not wild-caught but are farm-raised (aquaculture) where they ingest soy, corn, and processed grain. The fish are not eating what they would normally have in the lake or ocean. Now the oils in those fish are not good for us anymore and become very inflammatory.

Eating healthy takes time and patience, like making the effort to go the store and buying the right food. There are many hidden gems you can find at grocery stores. For example, a grocery store may carry a dozen prepackaged salads that an officer could grab on the go, and they offer a decent variety as well as being a healthier choice than a fast-food trip.

Losing weight is an excellent way to begin a healthy lifestyle. I try to discover the different roadblocks to why officers are not losing weight. If someone wants to lose weight, they will have to look at a few different variables. This often includes modifying lifestyle, diet, and exercise routines.

What Constitutes a Healthy Diet?

For diet, I recommend eating a lot of natural items like fruits and vegetables. However there should be a 2:1 ratio of vegetables to fruit. I also recommend an anti-inflammatory diet that incorporates the Mediterranean diet, which includes eating lean protein, fresh fish, olive oil, and clean produce along with a Paleo diet.

The Paleo diet involves only eating natural food, which means nothing that is mass-produced or processed, and usually not much that comes in cans, bags, or boxes. The most basic Paleo concept is, if you couldn't eat it "back in the day" when our society was a hunter-gatherer state, that food is probably not good for us. For weight loss, it is important to stick to the basics and enjoy more protein and less sugar. I recommend protein in the morning and more carbohydrate later in the day. Having more fish, lean meat, tree nuts, fruits, vegetables, and eggs would be a great start for most people.

The biggest culprit is the amount of sugar in many products that we consume and the regulation of these products in our country. Not everything advertised as healthy actually is healthy, and as Americans, our diet is loaded with way too much sugar. Many ingredients in the food we eat have high concentrations of fructose, corn syrup, preservatives, and food dyes along with genetically modified organisms (GMOs) that can have harmful effects on the human body.

Sugar

Eating the correct food in the morning is critical to starting the day off right. When we wake up, we should wake up hungry. If a person doesn't wake up hungry in the morning, something may be wrong with their metabolism. We help a lot of officers get their metabolism working again. Every individual is different, but there are enough similarities that indicate we should not consume a lot of sugar in the morning. Basically, everything we eat traditionally for breakfast in this country is terrible for us. Cereal and milk, pancakes and syrup, Pop-Tarts, toast, muffins, bagels, orange juice, donuts to name a few items, and the list goes on.

When a person consumes sugar in the morning, their blood sugar shoots up quickly. The body responds by lowering the blood sugar back down by secreting insulin into the bloodstream. What happens is the body loses control for the rest of the day, and that person actually loses the ability to regulate their blood sugar. It will cause peaks and valleys of blood sugar in their bloodstream, which is one of the things I test for in my office. This test is called *a hemoglobin A1C* test. When sugar rises too high to quickly for the body to control, there is a reaction that occurs that tacks sugar onto the person's red blood cells. With this test, we can help determine a person's risk for diabetes and cardiovascular disease. Less sugar, few carbohydrates, and more protein will generally work for people to become healthier.

Coffee

Another issue I see is coffee. Officers are known to drink many cups of coffee a day along with energy drinks and other stimulants. One thing that could be a problematic pattern for police officers who are worn down is using coffee for energy and a stimulant to stay awake until their shift ends. Coffee beans are harvested in a very hot climate, and they are very dirty. When the beans are in transport, fungus often grows all over them, and they form a toxic substance called *aflotoxin*, which can have a detrimental effect on the body. The coffee beans are often covered in pesticides and other toxins as well. Some studies say that coffee is healthy to drink, but I think coffee is really a toxic soup, and not that great for us to drink unless we go out of our way to get a trusted organic source.

Dieting

A problem I see with weight loss among police officers is that they may lose twenty pounds and then gain that right back—and more. Losing weight is a slow, steady process. Officers have to keep working at it every day. When an officer finds out they have high cholesterol, they should ask why, and not be happy with taking pills for the rest of their lives. We have officers saying they feel great, but when they come in they are taking six different medications. In their minds, they think they are healthy and they think everything is great and that their doctor is on top of things. I look at this officer, and although they may feel fine, their body on the inside is being held together by duct tape. Not all medications are bad; in fact some are lifesaving, but using them to cover a problem that otherwise could be solved by a lifestyle change never leads to good health in the long term.

I wish our system was more driven toward wellness and preventive care. We would have more officers who are healthier and less dependent on higher levels of intervention as they get older. My goal is to help every police officer I see who is in chronic pain to get healthy. We will teach them that staying healthy is a process. Why should they wait until they are sick? Officers need to change their lifestyles through diet and exercise and overall wellness. They would live longer and healthier lives.

Vickie Poklop agrees that getting police officers to eat healthy every day is quite a challenge, unless they are committed to packing healthy snacks and meals for every shift.

Unfortunately, it is part of the police culture to eat on the run, as officers have a limited lunch time and are often patrolling the streets and grabbing food to go: hot dogs, hamburgers, french fries, beef sandwiches, pizza, and a soda. These fast-food items may taste good but they do not provide the body and brain with optimal fuel. As a result, the food can make these officers feel sluggish, tired, and crabby. Even worse, they will still be hungry because they are not giving their body the proper nutrients they need.

Police departments do not have budgets that provide their officers with bowls of fruit, fresh veggie sticks, healthy snacks, or food of any kind for them at work. It becomes incumbent on the police officer to be dedicated to ensuring they eat nutritionally well all day long. It is one more responsibility to add to the seemingly endless growing list of tasks that each officer must accomplish each shift. Ensuring an officer's well-being, keeping their energy up and vibrant, comes down to healthy eating, getting enough rest, having meaningful relationships, and taking good care of their mental health. It is important that these officers also do physical activities and take the time to slow down and meditate and be mindful. For many police officers, the question is how. That sounds great, but how are they going to do that? Because that is the other real part of it: these officers have families, kids, side jobs, court, they are running here, there, and everywhere.

Getting Proper Sleep

As many young rookies will soon find out, the midnight shift is often the first shift they will experience in law enforcement. Officers with more time on the job often prefer and bid for the day or afternoon shift if possible.

I remember working midnights and always feeling tired. I could not get the proper rest I needed and was always catnapping during the day. I was cranky and on edge. I could feel that I was not as patient as I normally would be and could feel my attitude and demeanor were questionable at times. I was irritable at home and could not focus on simple tasks without continuously nodding off. No one explained any of this out of the academy. Tenured officers tried to give us advice about what worked and what didn't for them to get more sleep. One of the happiest days of my career when I was told that I would be on afternoons with a friend of mine from the academy.

Steve James, PhD, a research specialist in sleep deprivation, has suggestions for making sure officers get sufficient and quality sleep.

> For officers to get the best sleep at night, I recommend cold, dark, and quiet. Sixty-five degrees Fahrenheit is often the sweet spot temperature-wise to get a good night's sleep. A person's core drops when they go to sleep. They are helping their body out when they sleep in a cold environment. Keep the bedroom as dark as possible. An officer who is working the graveyard shift and trying to sleep in the morning should invest in blackout blinds. It will probably be the best investment they can make. Loud barking or sirens from ambulances that pass by can disturb you and pull you out of sleep too soon. Because of the various loud noises in the city, it is important to have a quiet environment, and it may be good to learn to sleep with

earplugs in. The other thing is to take technology out of the bedroom. There should not be a TV on the wall, no computer or iPad brought into the room, and try not to have a phone in the bedroom unless you are on call. If a person wakes up at night and sees a text message or email, they may soon engage in other emails or messages. Do not use a cell phones as an alarm; invest in an inexpensive alarm clock. It is important to limit technology, and to stop using handheld devices thirty minutes before going to bed because the light goes straight into your eyes at a close range. If you want to watch TV, watch it on a regular television set, not on a handheld device, and sit farther away from that light source.

It is important to listen to your body. Dr. William Dement, in his book *The Promise of Sleep,* makes this analogy about sleep. Think about when a person wakes up in the morning, and they imagine putting on a backpack. For every hour they are awake, they put a brick in that backpack. Most people who work nine to five are awake sixteen hours and get eight hours of sleep. So by the end of the day, they have sixteen bricks in their backpack. That is what we call their sleep debt or their homeostatic pressure to sleep. As we sleep, we take two bricks out of that backpack per hour, and we will start the day with an empty backpack. That is what a normal adult should sleep, but if they are sleeping less, they are adding extra bricks into their backpack. They cannot sleep long enough to repay the sleep debt they have accumulated. These are the problems that officers often experience working the graveyard shift. These bricks are the homeostatic pressure to sleep. It builds as we are awake and dissipates as we sleep.

Sleep is so important for officers to stay sharp on the street and emotionally healthy as well. Sleep hygiene classes should complement wellness classes offered in the police academy. I believe there should be annual and mandatory classes regarding sleep hygiene at the police academy.

A few simple sleep hygiene tips that may improve sleep:

- Make sure your bedroom is dark and cool when going to bed.
- Have a routine, going to bed and waking at the same time if possible.
- Drinking a warm, decaffeinated beverage may help relax you before retiring to bed.
- Limit TV and screens thirty minutes prior to going to bed.
- Invest in a very good mattress.
- Try meditation, yoga, or reading a book to relax before bed.

ALTERNATIVE MEDICAL TREATMENT OPTIONS

The term *alternative medicine* "describes medical treatments that are used instead of traditional (mainstream) therapies. Some people also refer to it as 'integrative,' or 'complementary' medicine … The definition changes as doctors test and move more of them into the mainstream."[13]

Acupuncture

The three main objectives of acupuncture are to relieve pain, strengthen the immune system, and, most importantly, balance and integrate the functions of the body's organs with one another.

Dr. Antonio F. Pugliese from Driven Wellness Acupuncture explains:

> Acupuncture is an ancient Chinese method of treatment that has been used for over 5,000 years. It is considered one of the oldest forms of medical treatment. Acupuncture typically incorporates the traditional use of very fine and flexible needles that are selectively placed on the body. The needles help to increase the blood flow and neuron impulse to the brain to alleviate issues that need

---

[13] https://www.webmd.com/balance/guide/what-is-alternative-medicine#1

to be corrected or adjusted. Acupuncture effectively and safely balances the chemicals in the brain with no negative side effects.

I have treated many police officers for physical ailments along with emotional concerns like stress, anxiety, and depression. Police officers have an extremely dangerous job and are constantly bombarded by stress. Cortisol, which is a stress hormone, is constantly being secreted into the bloodstream. The cortisol hormone first affects the body, then affects the brain. Because of the stress that officers endure, they often have higher levels of cortisol in their system.

The problem is police officers do not take care of themselves as well as they should. They often seek out immediate gratification, and they indulge by eating fast food because of their hurried lunch schedule. Because of this, many officers have a tendency to have larger waists and are at a risk factor for heart disease. Both are very common issues that many officers experience. The weight builds up around an officer's stomach area, and heart attacks are often near the top four or five categories of police-related deaths. In my opinion, it should be mandatory that every policeman receive acupuncture.

A recent six-week study done by John Allen, PhD, from the University of Arizona revealed that patients given acupuncture experienced a 43% reduction in depression-like symptoms. After acupuncture treatment, more than half of the patients no longer met the criteria for clinical depression.

It is important to note that acupuncture is just as effective as antidepressants and psychotherapy. It is extremely important to go to a licensed acupuncturist with a designation of LAC, which indicates they have studied acupuncture for six to eight years. LAC is the highest level of acupuncture a person can achieve.

Tony Bertuca is a former NFL football player who suffered from concussions for many years. After visiting many doctors and suffering from issues like short-term memory loss and headaches, a close friend mentioned that acupuncture might help. After doing some research, Tony decided to visit Dr. Pugliese.

> I was very skeptical at first because I did not know that much about acupuncture, and I had success after a few treatments. My energy picked up, my memory was getting better, and I felt less pain in my back and in my shoulder area. Dr. Pugliese was really making a difference in my life. I started doing memory exercises along with my weekly visits. I look forward to every session and I am truly an advocate of acupuncture and how it truly improved my life.

Meditation and Breathing Exercises

Everyone has their own approach and technique to relaxing and staying calm. Many individuals relax and diminish stress through meditation. Meditation and becoming calm and relaxed are all about breathing.

Breathing to Relax. When a person seems anxious and exited, someone may instruct them to "take a deep breath," which is a natural way to calm down and relax. Breathing slowly will also help that person strengthen their concentration.

Vickie Poklop says,

> There are simple things that everybody can do every day to help them relax. One of the biggest tricks to relaxing is to become aware of your breath. We breathe automatically and unconsciously. When we become aware of our breath, we can settle our nervous system. The first thing to notice is if you are breathing in for the same amount of time that you are breathing out in the same amount of time. There should be an equal balance to the in and out breaths. But often when we are stressed, our in-breaths are shallow. Shallow in and shallow out. That is a cue that we are stressed. To correct this, simply focus on taking in a deep breath that fills your lungs. Hold it for a couple seconds and then release it. Next, consciously breathe in for as many seconds as

you breathe out. If you can remember to do this once a day, you will notice that your nervous system will calm down. Use this useful tool any time during the day when you are feeling stressed. Police officers can do this in their vehicles, during roll call, in the courthouse, at home. It's a simple and effective coping skill that can be employed anywhere.

Meditation to Relax. Most people meditate in a quiet place by themselves often focusing on serenity and peacefulness when they find the time or need to relax.

My wife, Debbie, meditates when she first gets up in the morning. She closes her eyes, taking slow breaths that start to relax her mind. Often when she meditates, she concentrates on herself at that moment. Meditation helps her start her day with a calm routine. Debbie feels that meditation helps a person set themselves apart from the noise and the distraction of a busy schedule by being mindful in the present moment.

Hyun Kim of Naperville Meditation Center loves to share the benefits of meditation.

> Surely, we all see the world through our own thoughts including police officers, and vice versa. We are blinded by our own experiences. Therefore, it is easy to blame others, and it is very difficult to understand each other because everyone has their own set of filters through which they view someone else's life experience. We must first try to work on changing ourselves. I'm not here to influence others as an expert, but rather to connect with people who are searching to share in meditation.
>
> Meditation helped to open my eyes and has changed my life as a result. Meditation is a wonderful tool to not only reduce stress, anxiety, and fear, but also to become relaxed and to find your true identity. As a person meditates longer, they can discover the purpose of life, and an enlightenment that finds God and truth within, which is the ultimate goal. There are so many different types of meditation that can be used depending on a person's intention.

Due to [the coronavirus] pandemic, there has been much confusion in the world. We may wonder what is happening in the world right now. Why are we living this way? Through these difficult times, we see the fragility and the futility of human life and how quick it can end. A person can be here one day and gone the next. We are not really promised life.

So, first ask yourself, "Am I meditating to get away from my unwanted stress and emotions, or am I meditating to become complete, to move closer to my true values and honoring myself?" Many people practice meditation to control and calm their minds so they can be present in the moment, which has many benefits. Many people struggle to control their minds without knowing why. This causes anxiety, insomnia, heartache, and physical illness as well.

The mind they are struggling with and want to control is an illusion that happens only in their head through their life experience. Because our body operates the same as a camera, everything we see, smell, say, hear, and feel is sensationally and emotionally imprinted into our brain as a picture. We are attached to our experience and the memories in our mind, and we find ourselves trapped within our own mind, unable to free ourselves. This is why humans are incomplete. In meditation, awakening and awareness (mindfulness) mean to realize that this is a false illusion. Therefore, all the anxieties, fear, and worry are not an actuality.

Neuroscientist Professor Patrick Cavanagh from Dartmouth College says, "It's really important to understand we're not seeing reality. We're seeing a story that's being created for us. ... The brain also unconsciously bends our perception of reality to meet our desires or expectations. And they fill in gaps using our past experiences."[14] Meditation is a great tool to be free from the burden in our life. It is a tool to help navigate us toward total well-being

---

[14] https://www.vox.com/science-and-health/20978285/optical-illusion-science-humility-reality-polarization

in our daily life and to be enlightened to God and truth within. The root cause of our agony is the fear of the unknown and meditation will be help us experience true love and compassion in total harmony with ourselves.

Hypnosis and Hypnotherapy

Carol Henderson, a clinical hypnotherapist and certified emotional freedom techniques (EFT) practitioner, suggests hypnosis is a good way to heal the stressful events we all have in life.

Hypnosis is a difference in a person's awareness and perceptions. Some people say that it is a different state of consciousness from being fully awake and alert, that it is similar to daydreaming. We all go through a hypnotic state when we wake up in the morning, and also as we fall asleep at night. It is a state where a person is aware but not thinking too much.

Being in a trance is somewhat misunderstood. To think about something that happened in the past, a person has to go into a quick trance to access that information. For example, if I asked what your high school graduation was like, you have to access that memory from the subconscious mind where all those memories are stored. It is a natural process. "Highway hypnosis" is another example of a trance we all experience. This term describes someone who is driving and awake but misses their turnoff because they were deep in an awake trance.

The hypnotist cannot make someone go into a trance, but instead gently guides them by having them use their imagination to pretend they are in a beautiful, tranquil place, or that they are gradually relaxing their entire body one part at a time. Hypnosis is similar to meditation, where a person's mind becomes calmer. Some people feel they can't meditate because they can't quiet their mind, but in hypnosis, a person has the same benefits as with meditation, but they don't have to stop thinking, and they have the added bonus of hypnotic suggestions that can help them change their habits and feelings and heal the past.

In these troubling times, many people are in a constant flight, fight, or freeze mode. They might be constantly anxious and worried about what is going to happen next. This is an undesirable state for both the body and the mind. The body stays tense even while they are sleeping. Hypnosis can teach a person's body to relax. When they are in hypnosis, their heart rate slows down, their breathing slows, and their blood pressure goes down or regulates so that it is just right. When a person is relaxed, the body can heal itself from physical as well as emotional illness.

Traumatic events in the past keep us stuck and unhappy in the present. The emotions from these events can be neutralized by hypnosis or emotional freedom techniques (EFT). No matter how traumatic an event was, it is not happening now, and can be healed. The person may forgive themselves and others for the mistakes they have made. This is easy with these techniques. This helps the person move forward with no lingering shame, guilt, anger, disappointment, or fear.

Vickie Poklop has also been certified in hypnotherapy since 2015.

Hypnotherapy is a healing modality where we are able to work with the subconscious mind; I teach people how to turn down the dial on their reactions and their emotions. We are able to access a part of the brain that is a little calmer and not so reactive. In hypnotherapy, we can teach clients how to monitor their emotions and to release the charge they are getting from the experience so it is not so disruptive to them. This puts people in a calmer state so their brain waves are calmer. In a trance state, we can work on traumas big or small that are upsetting, like an argument with our partner that left us wounded, or something we said to our kids that day that we were not proud of, the big and small wounds that take up room in our bodies. Through hypnotherapy, we teach people to let go of that emotional charge, the anxiety, fear, guilt, anger, shame, sadness, or whatever the feelings may be, so that they are feeling free of unnecessary emotional baggage.

Emotional Freedom Techniques (EFTs)

Carol Henderson explains that EFT is a technique unlike any other you might be familiar with.

> With EFT, a person can heal feelings, memories, and thoughts by tapping with their fingertips on acupuncture points while repeating a phrase designed to bring up the feelings and neutralize them. This technique is being used on returning military personnel as well as during natural disasters in all parts of the world. It has been shown in trials to be more effective than other therapies for people who have been through severe trauma, such as hurricanes or tsunamis or earthquakes. The tapping on the acupuncture points soothes the amygdala, the fear center in the brain. This technique allows someone to think of the traumatic event and feel OK, calm, and peaceful. The person feels better about themself and is able to view the future with hope and excitement.
>
> EFT can be used for phobias, too. It neutralizes the fears. It can be used for eliminating resentment, feelings of inadequacy, grief, jealousy. or any other uncomfortable feelings. This technique is good for removing cravings for food or cigarettes, or the desire to do something else that is dangerous or unhealthy.
>
> It is an easy technique to learn, and people can easily do it themselves. A person can learn EFT for free from the internet. Some people say it is better to learn it at first from a guide or EFT practitioner and then use it on themselves. As we get older, the traumas in our lives, if not released, stack up, creating more and more anxiety, stress, depression, and worse. The feelings associated with these traumatic events, or even regular everyday events that are undesirable, are intended to be felt and then released, but we were never taught that as children or as adults. By learning and

practicing EFT, we can weed out the origins of our discomfort and then we are free to feel happy, confident, even joyful with our lives. Our life hasn't changed, but the way we look at it has.

Yoga

Yoga is a spiritual practice that originated in ancient India and is rooted in Hindu scripture and belief. Yoga encourages health, relaxation, spirituality, and happiness. Yoga is often considered a calming technique that helps a person become aware of their body and fine-tune how they are feeling while strengthening their muscles through specific body postures. It focuses on self-awareness and contributes to a person's mindfulness, love, and self-kindness. The guided and directed breathing exercises often help a person deal with daily stress. It provides the many needed tools to stay tranquil and calm in the anxiety and apprehension that we experience in our everyday lives. Many people have said that yoga helped them self-reflect their inner strength and perseverance.

The nice thing about yoga is that it can be enjoyed at any age or body size. Many people who have attended yoga classes say it has improved their demeanor and elevated their mood. If a person has had a stressful day at work, yoga has rejuvenated their positive attitude.

Years back, if someone told a police officer that yoga was a great alternative for relieving stress, they might have frowned at the thought of attending a yoga class. Rugged manly police officers would never attend a yoga class. One older officer who I previously worked with said,

> Are you kidding me, years ago I wouldn't get caught dead going to a yoga class. My wife insisted that I go with her when I retired. I started gaining weight and I was crabby most of the time. I was bored, I missed the job, the comradery, and I have no real hobbies. I have to admit I was reluctant to go and made excuse after excuse every week. She gave me an ultimatum; we went together or else. Well, I was shocked how many men were in attendance. My fear soon evaporated, and I learned to breath, relax, exercise, and enjoy the class.

I can't believe it, but now I look forward to going to yoga class three times a week with my wife. We have met a few nice couples, and we recently started socializing with them outside of our yoga class. One guy is a retired sergeant, and the other guy was with the FBI. Both said the same thing: they are glad they both fought the stigma of going to a yoga class. We laugh about it now.

I am happier than I have ever been, much calmer, I lost some weight, and my wife said that I am not as restless in bed. My suggestion to everyone in law enforcement, both male and female officers, is to at least try it; you will be amazed of the outcome. It changed my life in a positive way, and it probably saved my marriage because it did not look promising before yoga. It gives us something to do together. We laugh, have fun just like old times. That old police mentality took a toll on me and our marriage. I was stubborn and unforgiving. Yoga really changed my life, and I thank my wife often. My one and only regret is that I am sorry I didn't go to yoga sooner.

Dr. Eric Ramirez-Thompson says,

Yoga is a specific form of exercise. People can practice relaxation techniques, breathing, and things of that nature. We see physiological benefits from this. This is something that I actually teach to aspiring criminal justice professionals who are enrolled in my "Introduction to Criminal Justice" courses, and in criminology, we get into areas of the physical and physiological issues in dealing with police work and other related professionals.

Yoga is a non-traditional exercise with proven benefits, but many are inclined to resist such a recommended coping strategy because there is a "warrior" culture inextricably linked to police work. Yoga is perceived as an activity that doesn't build muscle, isn't deemed physically challenging, and has minimal physical benefits for men. Of course, "real men" would lift weights, so the officer who practices yoga risks being stigmatized.

The rejection of yoga and other alternative therapies is all deeply connected with police culture. Change and reform will require that those responsible for police training, educators, and our culture must integrate these activities into police training. As an educator, I believe it begins with us as we have the ability to set expectations for those entering the profession, deconstruct myths related to the warrior mentality, and emphasize the mind-body connection. I believe that emotional and physical self-care should be introduced in the police academy, so later in their careers when they hear about helpful coping strategies like yoga and meditation, it will not be the first time they are hearing about them.

Tai Chi

Chris Cinnamon, an exercise physiologist, lawyer, author, wellness expert, and head instructor at Chicago Tai Chi, explains another alternate form of exercise.

Tai chi originated as a martial art centuries ago in China and developed into a sophisticated, close-in fighting system. Today, tai chi is primarily practiced for its many proven health benefits. As an exercise, tai chi emphasizes low impact, whole-body movements that are easy on the joints, making it especially good for those with old injuries or arthritis. What's great about tai chi as an exercise is that it that works the whole body—muscles, joints, connective tissue, and the lymphatic, digestive, cardiovascular, and nervous systems. All of that combines to support vibrant health, even as we age.

A big difference between tai chi and most Western exercises is that tai chi emphasizes relaxing at ever deeper levels, rather than straining or pushing. This is especially beneficial for those that work in highly stressful occupations. Chronic stress has well-established pathological consequences. Tai chi helps a person feel where they are holding tension in the body and release it.

Among the mind and body exercises, tai chi is the most examined by Western medical researchers. The benefits of tai chi are well documented for reducing stress, improving mood, and improving, even eliminating, symptoms of many chronic conditions. Tai chi exercises the body, calms the mind, and helps people feel better.

I have to admit that when I first saw a few people doing tai chi in a park near my home, I was curious about the slow, orchestrated movements of these ten people, all in unison, each aware of every single movement of their body. Just like anything else, a person is more likely to criticize what they do not understand. I had never seen this before and was somewhat intrigued.

When they were done, I spoke to a peaceful and gentle man named Mr. Chen about their dedication to tai chi. Mr. Chen explained that tai chi incorporates slow, deliberate, and mindful breaths, and that he has been doing tai chi most of his life. He shared that he looks forward to his daily sessions with his friends. They have developed a strong bond, and his group has expanded in a short time. I told Mr. Chen about my reluctance to trying something new.

Mr. Chen explained the benefits of the slow, circular movements of tai chi, and how the exercise improves his overall strength as it relieves stress and improves his flexibility. He said his blood pressure has always been low, he has no arthritis pain, and he sleeps exceptionally well every night. He will be seventy-nine on his next birthday, and his doctor said he is amazingly healthy. He attributes his good health, calmness, and good fortune all to tai chi.

Qigong

Qigong is similar to tai chi, and it is also considered an ancient Chinese exercise. Qigong incorporates regulated breathing along with precise movement that has been known to help a person's balance, equilibrium, and flexibility. Qigong exercises can have a positive effect on a person's mental and physical well-being.

Chris Cinnamon is also an expert in Qigong, and explains,

Qi is the Mandarin word for internal energy. *Gong* is the Mandarin word for practice. *Qigong* just means "energy practice." Qigong helps a person deeply relax and feel grounded and refreshed. Qigong involves exercises that are designed to promote health, longevity, balance, relaxation, and well-being.

Many traditions hold that energy, or qi, runs through the body. According to these traditions, to the extent that energy flows smoothly and strongly and in balance, we are healthy. To the extent that energy is blocked, stagnant, or weak, we are more susceptible to disease.

The qigong I teach involves low-impact exercises that promotes balance, circulation, and strength of a person's energy. Qigong is similar to tai chi because it is a low-impact exercise. Qigong relaxation techniques are designed to re-energize a person as they release chronic tension and refreshes their internal energy.

Reiki

The practice of Reiki focuses on healing, spirituality, and self-care. I first became aware of Reiki through my daughter Laura, who has risen to the Fourth Level Master Teacher in Reiki. As someone who has always been proactive about relaxation and meditation, she is an advocate of promoting a positive attitude for the mental health and well-being of her clients.

The word Reiki (pronounced RAY kee) is Japanese. *Rei* means "divine wisdom and divine guidance," and *Ki* means "universal life force energy."

She supports the five Reiki principles:

1. Just for today, I release angry thoughts and feelings.
2. Just for today, I release thoughts of worry.
3. Just for today, I am grateful for my many blessings.
4. Just for today, I practice expanding my consciousness.
5. Just for today, I am kind to all beings including myself.

Laura shares some of the many benefits of a Reiki session.

For an individual, Reiki is a holistic approach that encourages balance between an individual's mind and body. It is also important for a person's mental, emotional, spiritual, and physical well-being. It helps to clear any negative energy as it begins to balance a person's positive energy. It is a healing energy through the hands by just touching certain points or by remaining over certain areas of the body. It would help a police officer who is often in a high stress environment. They need to relax and have a release from this stress, and Reiki can benefit them in this way. A Reiki session can help the officer take away and dissolve any negative tension they are experiencing. Reiki is a hands-on relaxation method. It uses what is called a life force energy to assist in the balance of one's self.

Laura explains that a Reiki session can be done through distance healing—a phone session, Zoom, Facetime, or just having a picture of the person for the healer to look at and concentrate on. Reiki places a person in a state of calm. It is comparable to a person receiving a full-body massage. Reiki also releases toxins from a person's body. Laura has shared many examples of the positive effects of Reiki: it increases the immune system, relieves joint aches and pains, helps release pent-up stress, and generally helps individuals breathe and feel better. As a Reiki healer, she can actually feel the tension in a person's body, and all she asks for is the person to be open-minded when receiving the session.

Laura explains the seven chakras associated with Reiki.

Chakras are focused and concentrated on the energy centers of the body. A chakra helps to restore a person's balance; it also helps to reduce stress. A person's chakra can be overactive or underactive or spin faster or slower by what they think and feel. Chakras promote a person's physical, spiritual, and emotional well-being. Chakras are also represented by color; the size and brightness of each chakra is determined by an individual's energy level, physical condition, and spiritual development.

Laura revealed there are seven main chakras associated with Reiki. They are:

1. The Crown Chakra is associated with the color purple and it is most often thought of as being connected with God.
2. The Third-Eye Chakra is represented by a dark purplish-blue color. The third eye concentrates on a person's intuition or their awareness.
3. The Throat Chakra is characterized by the color blue. This chakra is associated a person voicing their opinion. It is what a person tells themselves or others.
4. The Heart Chakra is denoted by the color green. The heart Chakra deals with compassion or love for themselves or others.
5. The Solar Plexus Chakra is associated with the color yellow. This is the chakra of personal power, the way a person feels about themselves, their ego, and what they tell themselves.
6. The Sacral Chakra is represented by the color orange. The sacral chakra is often associated with a person's emotional, passionate, and sexual feelings. This chakra also affects a person's creative life along with their financial life.
7. The Root Chakra is associated with the color red. This chakra represents being grounded and a person's physical stability.

My daughter Laura asked me if I was open to a Reiki session. I approached the hour-long session with optimism, hoping to experience the tranquility, balance, and harmony of this experience. She said as a trained Reiki Master, she uses the technique of placing her hands over a person's body to transfer positive energy to a specific area. She clarified that this type of healing enables relaxation, and it will enhance a person's emotional well-being. Laura has mentioned that many of her clients have said they feel more relaxed and had a more restful sleep after a Reiki session.

I began my session on a late Sunday morning. Laura instructed me to relax, close my eyes, and take a few deep breaths, and she wanted me to activate my energy. Laura asked me to let the healing of her hands flow throughout my body, and explained:

> Various people feel different things when I am doing Reiki on them. Some of my clients have expressed a slight tingling sensation, warmth, positive energy, or some have felt nothing at all. A majority of my clients feel peace and calm, and many of my clients are so relaxed that they often fall into a deep sleep.

Needless to say, I fell into a deep sleep. Laura said I even snored the first ten minutes of the session. When my session was over, I felt like I'd slept for ten hours. I was very relaxed, and my mind was in a calm state, no tension or stress.

Laura reiterated that Reiki works on the body, mind, and spirit. She believes Reiki can also reduce arthritic pain and promote healing. Reiki can also help with depression and being more aware of how to deal with unexpressed feelings, emotions, or thoughts that may have been suppressed due to fear or embarrassment. Laura believes being "open" to healing through the hands of Reiki's healing energy can promote a healthy and happy life. "Reiki allows anyone to tap into their true, higher self," she says.

I have had a few Reiki sessions with my daughter's healing hands since my first session, and each time I felt calm, tranquil, and serene. Reiki is a great and wonderful experience that I highly recommend for my colleagues in law enforcement.

Neurobiofeedback (NBF)

Dr. Phil Epstein (who I refer to as the original Dr. Phil) was instrumental in developing this unique procedure over the past twenty-five years of research. Dr. Epstein is a psychiatrist and a Fulbright Scholar whose specialty is brain investigations. Over the years, he was able to develop a program to look at the brain in three different ways; magnetic resonance imaging (MRI) to see structure and diseases of the brain, quantitative electroencephalogram (QEEG) shows the function of the brain, displaying over-and under-activity in regions of the brain, and the single-photon emission computerized tomography (SPECT) scan to observe blood flow, oxygen, and glucose throughout the brain, and view any type of excess or restrictions in flow. A neurobiofeedback session can see where the dysfunction and depression are coming from.

> Neurobiofeedback is a technique in which people are trained to improve their health by using signals from their own bodies. We use biofeedback successfully on a daily basis to help a wide variety of problems. We can help police officers with anxiety learn to be able to relax. Neurobiofeedback training can alter the electrical activity in the brain and hence change the problematic symptoms. We look at the gateway to the subconscious because we live to a great extent in our subconscious mind.

Neurobiofeedback training presents the user with real-time feedback on the brainwaves within the brain. I had a neurobiofeedback session given to me by neurobiofeedback coach Ed Epstein (no relation to Phil Epstein), who placed a headband across my forehead that contained three electrodes. I was able to view my live brainwave activity in that moment. My brainwaves activity was correlated to bars and graphs. Each positive and negative stimulus was displayed on the screen. Ed explained that he concentrates on the research side of the session. Anxiousness, being startled, or feeling relaxed will each be displayed differently on the computer screen.

His team tries to find the best approach to help their clients. Ed showed me how to relax my brainwaves. I was directed to say the word "peace" as I slowly inhaled, and when I exhaled I would say the word "calm." After five minutes of actually experiencing the emotions and feelings of the words of peace and calm, I was able to see just saying those words made a calming difference in my brainwave portrait.

Ed Epstein explained a bit more.

> There's a saying in scripture, "The peace I give to you; … let your heart not be troubled. … "[15] There is value to the power in words. Self-encouragement, no matter what the circumstances are, can

---

[15] John 14:27 (NKJV)

bring you back to a well-balanced area of your spirit, thoughts, and emotions. Give officers encouragement that there is another option to the solution. When we start to learn the patterns of certain brainwaves, we can determine a course of action to help them. We want to get to know who that person is from another perspective.

The process is about transforming yourself into present-time awareness, not changing yourself. If an officer is constantly dealing with a bad situation, we can help them learn to alter their perspective in a positive manner. We give our clients a different way to look at life, and it gives them hope, help, and direction. We do our best to help them get on track. We help them take control of their brain, not letting the brain control them. Behavior modification teaches them how to reset and regulate their actions. Whether overactive or underactive, the brain actually has a blueprint pattern of what goes on. We have to regulate the heart first before the brain will work. We have a fit-for-duty evaluation process to help an officer who may have experienced a traumatic experience. I am happy to say about 75–80% of officers will be able to go back to their law enforcement jobs.

Eye Movement Desensitization and Reprocessing (EMDR)

Another tool used to help people deal with traumatic events they've experienced is eye movement desensitization and reprocessing, known as EMDR. It is a unique therapy for individuals who experience PTSD, panic attacks, depression, and/or anxiety, and has been beneficial to many troubled individuals over the past twenty-five years.

This form of treatment was initially devised to ease the anguish and torment that was associated with traumatic memories. The human mind is not equipped to handle large amounts of trauma, so it protects itself by blocking out the bad experiences from the person's memory. EMDR is a safe way to bring out a disturbing situation that uses different techniques to disrupt brain patterns. Performed in conjunction with counseling, EMDR enables a person to reprocess the right and left brain, and how they think about and process traumatic events they have experienced. This particular therapy focuses on three things: past memories when the trauma first occurred, present issues related to that trauma, and strategizing for a more positive coping approach for the future.

First, the therapist helps the client relax their mind. The therapist then incorporates a bilateral movement that may include tapping the client's arm or moving their hands back and forth in front of their client's field of vison, as the client discusses the distressing incident at the same time. The person relives their past traumatic experience while they are focusing on the therapist's present stimulation. EDMR therapy has helped numerous people finally process their past disturbing experiences and help them heal their minds.

Cognitive Behavioral Therapy (CBT)

Police psychologist Dr. Marla Friedman says CBT encourages patients to focus on the present rather than the past. It examines an officer's current problems regardless of when those problems originated.

> CBT is one of the most widely effective forms of therapy for treating psychological conditions that include panic attacks, depression, and general anxiety. It can also benefit and improve an officer's relationships and family problems. CBT is used to help patients process traumatic memories, unbearable feelings, and intrusive thoughts that are common when a person suffers from post-traumatic stress injury. This form of therapy can also help people who suffer from intense stress resulting from the pressure of their job or problems within their personal life. It is a miracle in restoring officers to a healthy way of functioning again so they are fit for duty.

I believe police departments across the nation need to invest in their officers more, especially when it comes to their emotional well-being. It is time for police administrations throughout the country to take positive initiatives with their officers. Classes that emphasize wellness would benefit many officers who may be struggling at this present moment. Such classes could be in stress management, nutrition, sleep hygiene, couple counseling, meditation and breathing, finance, retirement planning, and a variety of other subjects. Especially important is offering mental health check-ins without any chance of it affecting the status of their jobs. Let's eliminate any stigma to receiving the help they may need without making them feel weak and embarrassed.

Beth Medina, the CEO of the Innocent Justice Foundation and the program director for SHIFT training, explains how her program can help.

> When we first started doing the Supporting Heroes in Mental Health Foundational Training program, we almost had to beg officers to attend this free, one-day training. It was challenging because police officers do not really trust mental health professionals. In law enforcement, mental health authorities are not called in unless there is a problem. These problems could be a fitness-for-duty question or assessing an officer for the job. Initially, it was not a positive relationship. When we go into training, we take a mental health specialist who has an understanding of the law enforcement culture and is an expert in trauma and we pair them with a law enforcement professional.
>
> This course is meant to be psycho-educational. It is meant to help officers help them understand what is happening in their bodies when they are in a trauma response. Officers get a lot of tactical training, forensic training, but this training can be instructive to officers to understand what is happening when they are engaged in a traumatic situation. It gives them a lot of power by first understanding how their bodies respond. They can structure a toolbox in a way to help them make a full follow-through on trauma response and not getting stuck in the trauma.
>
> Physiologically, what is happening in a trauma response? We talk about giving these officers tools they can use to help reset their bodies and their minds in these areas. We try to give these officers as many tools as possible to help mitigate the effects of the chronic exposure to trauma in these different areas in their relational lives

with others. We address vicarious trauma that can affect families and their entire police team. This training talks about those layers. This training also talks about exercise, nutrition, and breathing.

Breathing is one of the most important aspects of physiologically dealing with trauma recovery. Deep breathing will reconnect the brain and body back together quickly. This is a huge part of what we address in this training. Yoga and meditation is a great way for moderating breathing.

Practicing skills before there is a challenge is important to becoming resilient, which is the capacity to recover quickly from difficulties. Our training also identifies and incorporates skills the officer already has in place. We discuss why these skills are important: the more an officer intentionally chooses a response, the stronger their brain's neural pathway becomes. The goal is for their choice to become second nature—their go-to—when they face a challenging situation.

No officer would go on a search warrant without a Kevlar vest, their weapon, and everything they need to do their job. This training is like mental Kevlar for them. We know officers are going to encounter some of the most traumatic and stressful experiences a person can ever have to go through. We want to give them as much support as possible, and as many tools to recover from the trauma they experience and still do their job. Officers go into law enforcement with a mission-driven purpose, believing in helping their community and in justice. We have to support them in doing their job, and this training is how we provide that support.

Medina adds that social support is a key wellness factor.

Research done after 9/11 found that one quality of the most resilient people is the presence and use of social support. It is really important for our law enforcement professionals to have that sort of connection to their families and their social support systems.

Because when officers are "in challenge," social support is going to help these officers. Oftentimes when an officer is in trauma response and has an overload of traumatic stress, they do not often see it in themselves. It is the trusted people in their life who notice. If we have strong and personal relationships with trusted people, these are the individuals who often intervene and save lives.

Law enforcement professionals see the worst of the worst. It is like poison; they see it on a daily basis, they are in it, and what they do to prevent that from bleeding over into their families is sometimes pull away. Officers sometimes try to handle stress and trauma on their own or pull away and not share. They do not want to bring the trauma into their families and those they love the most. These officers will often isolate themselves even more than the job might isolate them. This can lead to many problems. It can lead to relationship problems in their marriages, it can lead to moms or dads not as connected to their kids. From the officer's point of view, they are trying to protect their child, but that is not how the child might envision it, and it might feel different for the child. Officers do not want what they see to bleed into their personal relationships.

An organization called 10-41, Incorporated, believes it is their mission to keep first responders "In Service" to their families and departments—physically, intellectually, emotionally, and spiritually. Reverend Timothy R. Perry, President of 10-41, Incorporated, shares the story about a phone call he received from an officer in crisis at 2:00 am. This officer had over fifteen years of experience in law enforcement.

We met soon after, and he showed signs of fatigue and anxiety. He sat at his workbench contemplating his future, and he knew about the stigma of asking for help. He was not going to show weakness. His plan was to show a face of steel as he pointed fingers at everyone but himself. The boundaries in his marriage had started to disappear, extramarital affairs in the end brought him nothing but pain. Performance issues at work had mounted, and his blue-line relationships had begun to weaken. He admitted it all came down to a bottle of liquor in one hand and a service revolver in the other. What once was a promising career right out of the academy became a decision to end it all. He told me, "I am five pounds away from ending this. Where does a person go when all of their decisions turn into pain?"

I was glad I answered that frightening call that morning. A broken-down officer who sought out the intervention he needed is now on a slow path to recovery. His dedication to change his life is an encouraging sign to a brighter future—something that he never realized could happen.

There are guiding principles that officers can manage and measure throughout their life. When challenges occur to any first responder on or off the job, they need to be addressed. Officers must strive to be resilient, and they must constantly look to improve their resilience. I recommend the science of neurobiofeedback (NBF) to the many officers I encounter in a serious and perplexing crisis. Leaders need the confidence knowing their officers will be able to manage their way through difficult times at work or at home. This technique will help to solve the emotional pain an officer is struggling with and most likely keep to themselves. With the use of NBF offered by noted psychiatrist Dr. Phil Epstein and biofeedback coach Ed Epstein, they are able to see how the brain is functioning when cops say "I'm fine." We can show them the level of anxiety, stress, and so much more from just in a few pictures of their brainwave activity.

HEALTHY COPING STRATEGIES FOR FINANCIAL WELLNESS

Mental health issues and physical fitness issues aren't the only factors to consider when discussing an officer's health. Any viable plan also needs to include financial wellness.

"Law enforcement professionals have the same concerns about buying a house, paying for college, paying down student loans, and retirement as the general population. Many departments choose to include financial counselling as part of their suite of mental health offerings for law enforcement personnel. It can lower stress for professionals and keep them inoculated from regulatory capture."[16]

Retired officer Coach Sok believes starting early to be financially independent is critical.

> For example, look at the police parking lot. A lot of young officers are driving expensive vehicles they want but do not need. How many of these young officers are living paycheck to paycheck? When they do not look at the whole picture, they might as well just shut off the lights, because they are not seeing anything as far as I am concerned. It is important for an officer to plan for something financially so they can support and sustain a purchase without cutting out other necessities. It is important to know how to budget, stay within the budget, invest for the future, and establish a child's college fund. I sometimes wonder how many police suicides result from financial overextension.

Doug Wyllie, who has authored more than 1,000 articles and tactical tips aimed at ensuring that police officers are safer and more successful on the streets, wrote an article in 2019 for *Police Magazine* titled "3 Keys for Financial Wellness for Police Officers."

> All too often police officers—particularly young officers just coming on the job—tend to get a little loose with their money, putting themselves in debt. The temptation to buy a new ATV, fishing boat, motorcycle, or other extravagance can be all-but unbearable when a rookie officer—whose only other job experience might be working at a retail store during college—sees those first few paychecks roll in.

---

[16] https://cops.usdoj.gov/html/dispatch/01-2020/reduce_stress.html

All too often, officers find themselves working second jobs out of necessity, or snapping up every available overtime shift just so they can pay the bills. Still others find that they've arrived at the moment when they can pull the pin and enter "retirement" only to find that retirement only means working a second career.[17]

STRIVE FOR BALANCE

I loved being a policeman so much that when I first came on the job, I would have volunteered to work an extra shift without hesitation. Wisdom changes a person over time. As officers, we need to take care of ourselves and live a well-balanced life. It is great being a police officer, but there is more to life than law enforcement. Our lives cannot be law enforcement 24/7, 7 days a week, 365 days a year. Once we leave the station, we need to leave the job there, especially when we go home to our families. Having outside activities is paramount to relieve the stress, anxiety, and tension we all have experienced doing police work.

Being a cop can be overwhelming, so we need to enjoy our time off, take the vacations, and get away from it all. We need to expand our horizons, practice mindfulness, and enjoy life. This goes for officers who are retired, too. It is not too late to do the things you enjoyed before or try new activities that will stimulate your mind and body. Being physically healthy and emotionally happy will lead to a long and prosperous life!

---

[17] https://www.policemag.com/511204/3-keys-to-financial-wellness-for-police-officers

—CHAPTER 11—

FINAL THOUGHTS AND
RECOMMENDATIONS FOR CHANGE

If one dream should fall and break into a thousand pieces,
never be afraid to pick one of those pieces up and begin again.
Flavia Weedn

I WANT TO do something a little different and unique for the last chapter and conclusion of my book. I want to share opinions and final thoughts of many of my fellow friends, officers, colleagues, therapists, clinicians, and experts in law enforcement about what should be done to enhance police wellness in our country. I believe each has a unique and important message that is needed to help all officers, both active and retired, enrich their emotional wellness and have a better life.

Final Thoughts from Dr. John Violanti, Author, Retired State Trooper, Expert and Researcher on Police Stress

> We need to teach officers how to cope. One good way is to enjoy life with their family. That is a great way to cope: exercise, play sports, do anything that is fun, and that will take their mind off the job for a little while. I think for some officers that is hard to

do, and it takes a lot of introspection to find within themselves the best way to cope with life. Officers need to "unplug" when they leave the job. Leave work behind.

They may ask, "What is the best way to deal with this job that I have to go out and deal with today?" Alcohol is not the way; it is maladaptive. The final maladaptive coping technique is suicide, and officers can get to that point through a bottle. I am not sure how to end this problem, but we have to depend on education to change behaviors and change attitudes. The influence of police culture is incredibly strong and difficult to change, but police work can be a rewarding profession if officers understand how it affects their lives and discover ways to deal with the job.

Final Thoughts from Chris Taliaferro, 29th Ward Alderman and Former Chicago Police Officer

We cannot let the cost of new mental wellness programs hinder us from helping the many devoted officers serving our city with courage and honor. They deserve respect from us when addressing emotional and psychological concerns. The first thing we need to do is hire the necessary and best police psychologists to address the issues that officers are facing in our department. We need to encourage our officers to get the help that they and their loved ones need without any repercussions. As officers, we spend a lot of time responding to calls and making sure that citizens are OK, but we often neglect ourselves. I believe it is important to never neglect yourself in the course of your duties as officers.

Final Thoughts from Matt May, Captain, Wake Forest (North Carolina) Police Department

I am thankful that my chief, Jeff Leonard, has created a culture for every rank below him that our department is willing to get our officers the help they may need. At the Wake Forest Police

Department, we want our officers to know that they are not alone, that we are a family. We spend more time with our police family than with our own families. We want to create a culture where an officer feels safe going to the command staff, a direct supervisor, or a fellow officer if they are struggling with the effects of trauma. Oftentimes, traumatized officers will believe the falsehood that they do not need help. They want to be courageous, want to be tough, want to be hard, want to believe that they are OK. All that is great on the street, and that will keep them alive. My question is, how's that working out for that officer and their personal life after a career in law enforcement?

Final Thoughts from Coach Bob Lindsey, Retired Police Officer and Speaker

The issue of police wellness is becoming a bigger and bigger issue in American law enforcement. Police are trained observers: they observe things, they observe events, and most importantly, they observe people. Then they are trained on how to handle people and events. What is not occurring is that we are not training police officers to observe themselves. Officers go out into the community every day to "Protect and Serve." I think that is pretty much a universal motto in the United States for law enforcement. I adhere to that motto; I agree with it, and I embrace it. In order for any officer to protect and serve the public, that officer, regardless of race or gender, has to have the willingness to take care of themself first.

Final Thoughts from Father Dan Brandt, Director of the Police Chaplain's Unit for the Chicago Police Department

My job and the job of those in my office is to remind our officers daily that they are doing God's work. They do not hear it nearly enough from their bosses, politicians, and the public. Officers often will either call me or one of our fellow chaplains seeking guidance and counseling because they know that what they say to us will always stay confidential. Confidentiality is very important to them. I would like to conclude with my thought with a verse from the Bible in Romans 13. It speaks about how God ordained sentinels, which is a term that was used 2000 years ago, and what we would call police officers today. Their work is ordained by God. It is not always pretty, where the sentinels carry out the work of God. It may cost them their lives, but it is God's ordained work. If they mess up and end a life doing this work, God will still smile on them.

Final Thoughts from Dr. Marla Friedman, Police Psychologist

When a person arrives as a recruit, they have already been through testing and evaluation. They are, in fact, mentally healthy. Look at them in years two, five, seven, fifteen, and so on, and they are no longer the person they were. These changes are more than the normal changes someone would expect from maturation and normal development or from life's wear and tear. The job itself has changed that officer, and usually in unhealthy ways.

Final Thoughts from Dr. Eric R. Ramirez-Thompson, Educator

We ultimately need to support a new era of police leadership with a more innovative view of the police profession and the importance of health, and this must permeate all elements and aspects of training. Police also need to find the balance between protector and enforcer, but to ultimately protect themselves first, not only physically, but also mentally and emotionally. Training is key and essential, and that begins through education.

Final Thoughts from Doug Monda, Founder of Survive First

The solution is that we have to change the way we train and do business, and it has to come from the top. If the administration does not buy into it, it is not going to work. That is the biggest issue that we have to deal with as officers today. We must change and introduce proper and different forms of training. Unfortunately, in our industry of law enforcement, depression, PTSD, and police suicide are the buzz words now. We are talking about them and introducing these terms into law enforcement daily. Cops out on the street have to have a sharp mind, then they have a sharp sword. If the officer's mind is sharp, their sword is going to be sharper. They are going to make better decisions if they are thinking clearly, and they will feel better physically and mentally. The greatest tool an officer can have in their duty belt is a sharp mind.

Final Thoughts from Dr. Luke Fairless, PsyD, Illinois Department of Corrections

No matter how open our administration is, they are sometimes at a loss to do anything in regards to emotional wellness because there is not enough research on the subject. There are just so many barriers, and anyone seeking treatment faces numerous obstacles in their correctional career. Law enforcement and public safety officers perhaps face some of the biggest silent barriers when trying to seek treatment for issues they may be experiencing. Whether the law enforcement culture is looking at its members as weak for seeking counseling, there is a need to stop the stigma of getting professional psychological intervention.

In the prisons in the rural areas of Illinois, correctional officers seeking help and getting the services needed can be quite difficult. Our officers are most often isolated from support networks outside of corrections. These correctional officers can easily fall into bad habits. They may begin to neglect their physical, mental, and emotional health. In the last ten years, these barriers have played a role regarding risk factors, mental health among inmates, and the likelihood of correctional officers experiencing a critical incident at work. With that being said, many prisons are in rural areas, and the context of seeking psychological help often becomes difficult because of barriers the correctional officers face.

Final Thoughts from Lieutenant Adrienne Gardner, Richmond (Virginia) Police Department

We have to teach emotional wellness and fight against the stigma of seeking help early on in the Academy and follow up with these officers throughout their careers. Our recruit training includes emotional wellness training that is explained and discussed by multiple people. We had one in-service training on police wellness, but we definitely need additional training. When is the next opportunity for our officers to receive this information again? It should not be a one-hit wonder, but we need to continually reinforce the vital material and information on police wellness to our officers. Over the years, our officers have become more mindful, and they are willing to speak to management when they see something that is emotionally affecting officers they work with. We had a female officer handling a murder scene investigation. A few of her fellow officers stepped up and said she was troubled by it, and they were concerned about her behavior and were reaching out on her behalf. Our department gave her some options to help her, and she was much better mentally and emotionally because of that needed intervention.

Final Thoughts from Lieutenant Frank Scarpa, Richmond (Virginia) Police Department

In-service training is a good way to get information on emotional wellness out to our officers. We want to make this training more of a staple beginning with recruit training, and then by continuously reinforcing it with in-service training every two years. Some of our veteran officers who have been working for ten to fifteen years are on the fence about getting help. We let them know that it's OK to ask for help and speak about what is bothering them at work or at home. That it is OK to speak to someone and get an issue off of their chest. I think that will go a long way with helping future officers by removing that stigma of seeking help for emotional issues.

Final Thoughts from Chris Scallon, Retired Sergeant with the Norfolk (Virginia) Police Department

I do many presentations throughout the country on the stress within law enforcement. Cops are not worried about themselves, but they are concerned about how people look at them, and that's the problem. If someone came to another officer and said, "I'm struggling," 100% of officers say yes, they would help them without a doubt. But ask them the question, "If you were struggling, would you reach out for help?" and maybe 10% of the people at my presentation would raise their hand. That's the problem: we are willing to help everybody, but we are not ready to help ourselves.

I got better when I stopped caring what other people thought and started focusing on how I get better. This did not come overnight, but it took me years and years of struggling and being embarrassed about it. It is our inability to process situations that we believe create shame, or that have us feeling shame. Once an individual puts aside how other people think about them, they can really begin to start healing. It really is that basic, but I was struggling for ten years through this stuff that was bothering me. No one cares if you are sick, just work on getting better. For me, the important thing is to understand why officers are struggling. It is really easy to tell someone what is wrong with them, but it is difficult to identify our own issues, and it's even harder to address those issues.

As someone who helps first responders and veterans, I can tell you that when they do address their issues, they never want someone to fix their problems, but they want help and a role in fixing their problems themselves. We need to establish a culture where obtaining help is the norm and we look out for each other, despite how awkward or uncomfortable we might feel.

Final Thoughts from Denise M. Coyle LMFT, CTS, Psychologist

We need education because every time that I have gone into a police or fire department and explained to them what happens after a traumatic event, they show concern. I reveal to them this is what a police officer or firefighter can expect their body and brain to do after a disturbing event. These are the signs they can look for; this is what is going to happen to them step by step; then the light bulb goes on, and recognition happens. I just normalized something to them that was foreign and had produced a lot of fear.

We help them realize that if we can identify a problem, we can take care of it. We feel that if we can educate officers about trauma, depression, and anxiety, we can save a lot of lives. When I get involved in an officer-involved shooting, I cannot talk to them about the events of the shooting. What I can do and what I find works well is telling them that this is what is going to happen within the next seventy-two hours. They are going to start feeling this in their body, this is what their brain is going to start doing, and this is what their sleep cycle is going to be like. The minute I normalize what they are going through and give them details of what to expect, they calm down. In the next seventy-two hours when they check in, the officer involved in the shooting will say, "Yeah I hit this stage, you were right about this part." It suddenly prevents the officer from going into that anxiety spiral of thinking they are going crazy, or thinking that something is wrong with them. This also prevents the officer from shutting down. They realize that we know what we are talking about and what they are going through. They start asking questions, was this also normal, will this also happen? It creates a dialogue from that moment forward that helps them through the trauma. So, we have to educate and present the details of how trauma, depression, and anxiety impact their body and their mind. We have to make this information accessible to first responders before, during, and after traumatic events. We have to stabilize their mind and body and give them the knowledge to become emotionally resilient.

Final Thoughts from John Marx, Retired Police Officer and Author

Looking at our profession today, we are suffering. Some of it we have brought on ourselves, some of it we have not. We need to make some changes. We have had wake-up calls in the past, and I just don't think that it made enough of a difference. I think that it is time to really take hold of our honorable profession and take it a step higher because we need to challenge ourselves to be better. I am such a strong believer in comprehensive wellness. I think we have not been training ourselves in the right way for so many years.

Look at the myriad of problems we have in our profession. From the outside looking in, we are being accused of excessive force, racial bias, or being too paramilitary. Look at issues about suicide, depression, post-traumatic stress disorder, issues with substance abuse, marital issues, and frustration issues. We get trained in the police academy and throughout our career about the overt dangers in law enforcement. The chances of us getting hurt, stabbed, or shot increase just from putting on our police uniform. I think because of that training, we have lost sight of some of the things that are really eating away at us from the inside out. Those issues are anger, depression, frustration, and suicide. Those, in my opinion, are symptoms of people who have not trained themselves to be healthy and well, and they have not been in an environment that has a support system that can keep them that way.

I often speak about the military model that has its purpose in law enforcement, such as uniforms, discipline, and authority. I encourage people to look at a sports model. Just take American pro football as an example. We spend all kinds of money finding amazing talent, and we put them out on the field. Watch one of these professionals get injured on the field, they drop down to the ground, and people rush out to help them. They hover over him, trying to find out what is wrong. If he is able to keep playing, they send him back into the game. If not, he is helped off the field to the sidelines. As the cameras continue to watch, they work to get him back into the game.

I am wondering why don't we consider our police professionals the same way as sports figures. Why aren't we making our police officers the best that they can be? Why are we not taking care of them, supporting them, and making sure they are fit to be in the "game"? Part of that responsibility lies with the officers themselves.

We are not looking at this the way we should. We are not looking at our profession as a profession. We are not looking at it as our life's calling. We do not hone our skills forever. We go to the academy, we learn some things, we gain experience out in the street, and we get annual training that takes the liability away from the department or agency. We are not developing ourselves in our true calling as masters of our craft that is policing. We have to start early, and we have to change the mindset and mentality to the idea that officers need to train themselves physically, mentally, emotionally, and spiritually every day. We need to be the best that we can be. When we start having challenges, we need to react to them immediately.

It is important that we change the mentality of our profession regarding the way that we sustain our officers. We need to help keep our officers in the "game." Policing, in my opinion, is the most noble calling on the planet, but it is also the most toxic. We just throw officers out on the street and expect them to deal with trauma and tragedy, day after day, and stay perfect and not be angry, and not be fearful, and not be immature, and not be a whole lot of things. We expect them to have the best reaction times, the best sense of compassion, and the best communication skills and the best decision-making skills, and yet we don't train them for any of those things. We need to make changes going forward.

Final Thoughts from Chaplain Al Lopez, Chicago Police Department

Police officers do not get that pat on the back or the thank you that they deserve. In the Bible, Romans 13, it says that sentinels (police officers) are the chosen, they are the peacemakers. Police officers are the barbed wire that stand between the sheep and the wolves. The Bible says evil runs around like a roaring lion looking for someone to devour. Police officers save lives just by being in uniform, getting out of their squad car, going into a store, or walking their beat. God bless our police officers, and may they never give up, may they never surrender. Blessed are they who are persecuted for the sake of righteousness, for theirs is the kingdom of heaven.

Final thoughts from Joe Gentile, Retired Police Officer and Hostage Negotiator

It is imperative for every police department or organization to have the resources available to every officer under their command. They need to have an outlet and the opportunity to address their issues. I had an uncle who died from suicide. He felt trapped and had nowhere to go, nowhere to turn, no outlet for help. My uncle was in construction, and his union did not have any resources available, mostly because it was frowned upon. If a person went for help, they were considered wimps. After all of the Crisis Intervention Team (CIT) training and hostage negotiations training, I know what is going on in the mind of an officer who is in crisis. It is important for the police union and the chaplains unit to always be in constant contact with our officers, to let them know that it is OK to get help without fear of retaliation. An officer's biggest fear is someone finding out, and they will be looked upon in a negative way. It's stressful.

It all plays on the officer. It is sad. Could we reach out to an officer who needs help? Can we see the signs? It is extremely important to get the help you need, not only for you, but for your family.

Final Thoughts from Coach Bruce Sok, Retired Police Officer and Speaker

I think wellness includes planning for the next chapter in an officer's life and to assist people looking down that road long before retirement. What is the next step? What am I going to be doing? What should I be thinking about to start preparing for retirement? The question of wellness is the total sum of these ideas. Occupation is one thing, but besides family, and if that officer does not have family and a circle of friends, what are their outlets? Do they have interests in other things? I tell the young cops, "What you do on the street is critical, but what you do off the job is going to have a major impact on how far you are going to go on this job. Don't confuse *what you do* with *who you are.* Don't get married to the job, but love what you do. When you go off duty, live life to the fullest; enjoy life. Don't be that person who is on the job 24-7, 365 days of the year, the cop who never goes off duty; that is not healthy."

They are going to get to a point when they pull the pin and become eligible for retirement. They stamp your police ID as a retired member, and they are going to walk you out that door, and the first thing that is going to hit you like a tsunami is, "What do I do now?" They know that they are going to miss the clowns, but not the circus. If that job as a police officer is all that they had, and it became the largest part of their life's focus, then there's not much going forward in their next chapter in life.

A police officer should plan financially for their retirement throughout their career, not just the last few years before they pull the pin and retire. It is important to be able to maintain a comfortable lifestyle. Total wellness is multidimensional and holistic. It requires career-life counseling with constant mental health services, wellness training, nutrition components, and financial planning. Alas, you can always tell young cops, but sometimes not much. I am not without hope, but hope is not a strategy for success. There's a lot of work to do.

Final thoughts from Carl Alaimo, PsyD, Retired Director and Chief Psychologist of Mental Health Services at Cermak Health Services of Cook County (Illinois)

One of the things that bothered me the most over my career was whenever the administration needed budget cuts, the first cuts were always to education and training. Then what usually happened simultaneously is we would see an onslaught of stress and suicide.

The administration will question how are they going to get the staff off the street. It is similar to a double-edged sword; it has to be done. I am an avid believer that most officers, whether it is law enforcement out in the street or our folks in the court system and corrections, are not working a 9 to 5 job. They may be on a rotating shift or on midnights, and this adds to their daily stress. Then when they have to pull somebody on the midnight shift and tell them they have training from 7:00 am to 3:00 pm, they really are turning that officer's world upside down. The reality is that we need to emphasize that training and education is the way to improve the lives of our officers.

The last thing in the world an officer wants to hear about is stress and psychology. The issue becomes, "OK, we agree, but what are you going to do for us to help us to relieve the stress on the job?" We say to them that their eating habits are off, their sleeping habits are off, they do not have extra free time, holidays or birthdays with their family. We explain the things that are stressors and educate them, then we turn them loose and we do not correct or further their education.

I think it really has to be from the top down. Whoever the top person is in charge has to make sure that the supervising staff is fully behind this initiative to make this work for the line staff. The brass and the leadership must figure out a way to incorporate education and training into their program. It has to be done if we are going to change the mortality rate of our line staff.

Final Thoughts from Rabbi Moshe Wolf, Police Chaplain for the Chicago Police Department

I am going to ask you a question. Have you ever been to a wedding?

Did you ever notice at a wedding that there are two types of people? There are people who dance in the middle of the dance floor, they twirl, they wave their hands and make funny dance moves, and then you have people who stand on the side who will say, "No I don't dance." I go over to them and ask them why they do not dance. "I can't dance," they'll answer. "People laugh at me, and I look funny." I tell them, "Please do not deprive yourself of the beautiful dance of life, because you think someone is going to laugh at you. Go out there and dance, go out there and sing and do your thing, go out there and be in the middle of the party. Don't worry about what other people think, go out there and live life and love life."

Sometimes we are afraid to do things, but why? Because people will laugh at us. So you are not going to run the marathon, so you are not going to the dance. I believe that everyone should enjoy the marathon, enjoy the dance, and do not let people steal the fact that you are human.

These are the two most important lessons in life that I think of when I attend a funeral.

Lesson #1: In life, people will experience pain and sorrow. It could be a divorce, an accident, a physical loss, loss of a limb, loss of eyesight, or loss of a spouse.

Don't feel the need to say something, but pay that grieving person a visit, go anyway, and be there for them in their time of need. Just say, "I am thinking about you, and I am keeping you in my prayers."

Lesson #2: No one is guaranteed tomorrow. Find something to laugh about each day, even if you have to look in the mirror. When a person goes through life's ups and downs and they tell me that God is their copilot. I tell them that if God is your copilot, switch seats.

Isn't it interesting in life that when we see somebody cry, what is the first thing that we say? "Be strong." What is wrong with somebody being able to cry? What is wrong with telling someone, "I am sorry for your pain." Isn't it interesting in life that if someone tells a good joke, does anyone say, "Don't laugh"? Go ahead and cry, it is good for the soul.

My Final Thoughts from the Author, Dr. Ron Rufo

I wrote this book for officers to take a good hard look at the life they have been living. It is my hope and dream that this book will inspire officers to sidestep the path that leads to despair and begin to follow the road to peace and happiness. Officers often deal with sadness and sorrow on a daily basis. Many officers are expected to just "suck it up." The only problem is that officers are human, not robots; they have feelings, and it is often difficult to just put those horrifying scenes out of their minds. Officers often suffer in silence, by themselves, not wanting to share past experiences that have begun to pile up like excess baggage. Officers are asked to go from one traumatic incidence to the next, without being able to process what they have just experienced. Supervisors need to step up and take officers who are on their team out of service for a while. This will give those officers a chance to regroup and process the severity of the incident. An officer is built up to be brave, strong, and unbreakable—but as human beings, we all have our breaking point.

There is no one size fits all when it comes to emotional wellness. I believe the best way for an officer to embrace emotional wellness is through a gradual transformation. No one likes drastic change, and police officers often lead that group. I believe three components are needed to sustain emotional wellness that will lead to lead a happier and healthier life. Those three components are physical, psychological, and spiritual wellness. I believe that each component intertwines with each other; leave out one of the three ingredients and it lacks balance.

Physical: We need to fuel the body with nutrients and healthy food. I like the saying that we need to eat to live, not live to eat. Many people have said they experience euphoria when they work out, exercise, run, or walk. It is also important to get the proper amount of rest so the body can function correctly.

Psychological: Police officers need to engage in a new way of thinking. Optimism should be their constant shadow. They need stress management techniques in their lives, which includes learning not to take home the problems they have experienced on the job, and taking a deep breath a few times a day to relax their minds and bodies. Officers need to seek and provide support for one another. They need to tune into their feelings when overwhelmed with stress. Most of all, they need to forgive, not only themselves but others. Holding on to a grudge does nothing but bring a person down. They need to be open to positive change and having a vision of what happiness is all about.

Spiritual: Officers need to take time to be alone and listen to their inner souls, and make peace within themselves. It helps to meditate and relax after a stressful encounter. They can nurture that inner spirit through yoga, Reiki, and other techniques to relax their mind and spiritual well-being.

I have seen many first responders suffer silently in pain, trying to figure in their minds how they can accept and deal with the emotional pain of the job. When a person breaks a leg, they get it repaired, no questions asked. No one would walk around with the pain from a broken leg. A police officer's emotional well-being is just as important. That stigma of being weak if they seek help must be buried once and for all. It is important to know that getting any form of mental help or therapy is what they need to heal any pain that they may be suffering or have suffered on the job as first responders. Officers are human, and they may need to talk to someone about the trauma they have encountered or witnessed on the job. They just can't carry the weight of those tragedies and misfortunes that weigh heavy on their shoulders. How much can the officer take before their emotional state is overwhelmed with frustration and depression? I compare an officer who is willing to express their feelings to someone who would like to cleanse their soul. Just this simple explanation is like having the weight of the world lifted off their shoulders.

When an officer is dealing with family issues, it is important for them to abandon the law enforcement persona they use on the street and leave the controlling attitude at the station. It is important to not be in cop mode or bring their job home. This drill takes practice, understanding, and patience. If a law enforcement officer takes their "controlling street attitude" home with them, it can cause many problems within the family.

I hope this book will gradually change the culture within every police department across the country. I truly feel that many police administrations should take better care of their officers. Here are a few of my suggestions that I believe would enhance wellness for a majority of police officers.

- More family days at the police academy
- Mandatory yearly nutrition classes
- Mandatory yearly sleep hygiene classes
- Mandatory yearly fitness tests and weight tests
- Mandatory yearly stress reduction and mental health check ups

Life has its many ups and downs, and it is important for officers to realize they are not alone when they experience pain, suffering, and anguish from the job. Taking care of their emotional well-being and getting needed help is paramount to a healthy life. Again, thank you and stay safe physically, mentally, but, most of all, emotionally.

To every officer in law enforcement, we need to carry our brothers and sisters when they need us, when they are down and out and feeling alone, desperate, and confused. Get involved, listen, and do your best to be a friend and be supportive of them, and never be judgmental. That is what police camaraderie is all about.

I would like to end this book with "A Police Officer's Prayer."

A Police Officer's Prayer
Lord, I ask for courage-
Courage to face and conquer my own fears ...
Courage to take me where others will not go ...
I ask strength-
Strength of body to protect others,
and strength of spirit to lead others ...
I ask for dedication-
Dedication to my job, to do it well,
Dedication to my community, to keep it safe ...
Give me, Lord, concern for those who trust me,
and compassion for those who need me ...
And please, Lord, through it all,
be at my side ...
Author Unknown[18]

Thank you for taking the time to read my book. I hope every day is filled with joy and laughter. Your emotional wellness is imperative and essential for a happy life. God bless!

Ron Rufo, EdD

---

[18] http://www.mdfallenofficers.org/police-and-st-michael.html

Thank you for reading *Breaking the Barriers: Changing the Way We Support the Physical and Mental Health of Police Officers.*

If you enjoyed reading this book, I respectfully ask for your honest review where you purchased it. Reviews help other readers decide which book to read next, and I would greatly appreciate yours.

If you have any questions or comments, or would like to learn more about me and the work I'm doing to help support police officers, please contact me at ronaldrufo@sbcglobal.net, LinkedIn, and join me on Facebook at facebook. com/RonRufo.

Other books by Ronald A. Rufo, EdD

Police Suicide: Is Police Culture Killing Our Officers?

Police and Profiling in the United States: Applying Theory to Criminal Investigations

Sexual Predators Amongst Us

RESOURCES

The only mistake you can make is not asking for help.
Sandeep Jauhar

When a police officer initiates a call to a crisis or suicide hotline, it is an urgent call that they need HELP at that very moment. A call not answered could be disastrous. It probably took that officer all that he had to pick up the phone and dial. There may not be a second chance at this point. The problem for a vast majority of officers is taking the initiative to even pick up their phone and ask for help.

This is an awkward place for them to be in. They are accustomed to giving help 100% of the time, not asking for help. Officers in a crisis situation will often reach out to an out-of-state crisis-and-suicide facility or hotline.

Regardless of the circumstances, knowing they *can* reach out for help is a message we all need to share. The following is a partial list of resources available to police officers.

Alcoholics Anonymous: A fellowship of men and women who share their experience, strength, and hope with each other that they may solve their common problem and help others to recover from alcoholism. The only requirement for membership is a desire to stop drinking. https://www.aa.org

Al-Anon and Alateen: Provides strength and hope for friends and families of problem drinkers. https://al-anon.org

Badge of Life: Provides comprehensive education and training to law enforcement about mental health and suicide prevention for officers and their families with a "Building A Better Cop" program. https://badgeoflife.org

Chateau Recovery Addiction and Treatment Center: A complex treatment transition support and a comprehensive assessment and testing family education support for PTSD, depression, and anxiety. 888-971-2928 | https://chateaurecovery.com

Concerns of Police Survivors (COPS): Various programs for police survivors for spouses, parents, siblings, teens, adult children, in-laws, and coworkers. 573-346-1414 | https://www.concernsofpolicesurvivors.org

CopLine: A not-for-profit 501(c)3 dedicated to serving active and retired law enforcement officers and their loved ones by providing confidential 24/7 trained retired officers for callers that are dealing with various stressors law enforcement careers encounter both on and off the job. Also able to assist with a referral to a culturally competent mental health professional. Calls answered by a retired active peer listener. All calls and emails are strictly 100% confidential. 1-800-267-5463 | www.copline.org/contact-us

CopsAlive: Provides information and strategies to help police officers successfully survive their careers. 303-940-041 | www.copsalive.com

Drug Dangers: Committed to providing information on a range of medications and medical devices that have serious complications. 888-584-0411 | https://www.drugdangers.com

Fellowship of Christian Peace Officers (FCO): A national ministry comprised of Christian men and women from all areas of criminal justice. 523-553-8806 | https://www.fcpo.org/www

First Responder Addiction Treatment (FRAT): Provides a complete range of services for alcoholism and drug dependency. 1-855-372-7435 | www.responderaddiction.com

Gamblers Anonymous: A fellowship of men and women who share their experience, strength, and hope with each other that they may solve their common problem and help others to recover from a gambling problem. The only requirement for membership is a desire to stop gambling. http://www.gamblersanonymous.org/ga/locations

Help Our Marriage: For married couples facing difficult challenges in their relationship. 800-470-2230 | www.helpourmarriage.org

International Critical Incident Stress Foundation: Provides leadership, education, training, consultation, and support services in comprehensive crisis intervention to emergency response professions. 410-750-9600 | www.icisf.org

Loving Outreach to Survivors of Suicide (LOSS): A program for adults and children, offered by Catholic Charities of the Archdiocese of Chicago. 312-655-7283 | www.catholiccharities.net/GetHelp/OurServices/Counseling/Loss.aspx

National Alliance on Mental Illness (NAMI): The nation's largest nonprofit grassroots mental health, advocacy, education, and support organization. NAMI is dedicated to building better lives for the millions of Americans affected by mental illness. www.nami.org/Home.

National Suicide Prevention Hotline: A national network of local crisis centers that provides free and confidential emotional support to people in suicidal crisis or emotional distress 24 hours a day, 7 days a week. 800-273-8255 | suicidepreventionlifeline.org

Officer Down Memorial Page: Nonprofit organization dedicated to honoring America's fallen law enforcement officers to preserve their memories and give friends, family, other officers, and citizens alike the opportunity to remember the fallen and honor their sacrifices. www.odmp.org/contact

Road Home Assistance Program: Provides mental health care and wellness to veterans of all eras, service members, and their families at no cost and regardless of discharge status, in any way possible. 312-942-8387 | https://roadhomeprogram.org/

Spirit of Blue: Dedicated to the enhancement of officer safety and vitality throughout the law enforcement community by promoting public awareness for their protection and fulfilling safety equipment and training needs. https://www.spiritofblue.org/about-the-foundation/contact-us/

St. Michaels House: A highly confidential inpatient and outpatient substance treatment center dedicated exclusively to the care of law enforcement officers. 847-813-3300 | https://www.amitahealth.org/careers/facilities/amita-health-holy-family-medical-center-des-plaines

Suicide.org: Suicide prevention, awareness, and support. Provides a listing of 24/7 Suicide Hotlines in each state. 1-800-SUICIDE (1-800-784-2433), 1-800-273-TALK(1-800 272-8255) | www suicide.org

The CORE Matters Project: A multidimensional classroom experience focusing on social emotional learning, empathy, and respect building instruction utilizing cooperative learning activities, role playing, classroom discussions, individual work, as well as physical activities. www.coremattersproject.com

Under the Shield: Provides support through confidential services, education, and awareness. 855-889-2348 | www.undertheshield.com

Violently Injured Police Officers: Provides peer support to law enforcement officers who have been seriously injured or have had to use deadly force in the line of duty. Provides support, information, and resources to these officers and their families to assist in the transition after suffering physical and emotional injuries. www.vipo911.org

Willow House: A nonprofit social service organization whose sole mission is to support children, families, schools, and communities who are coping with grief and the death of a loved one. 847 236-9300 | https://willowhouse.org

Contributors and Experts

Carl Alaimo, Sr., PsyD: Carl is the retired director and chief psychologist of Mental Health Services at Cermak Health Services of Cook County, Illinois.

Barbara Arkwright: Barbara is a Special Agent in Charge, Law Enforcement Division, Office of Enforcement and Compliance, Department of Motor Vehicles, Richmond Virginia.

Tony Barsano: Tony is currently a Chicago Police Officer with over twenty-five years of experience.

Roger Bay: Roger is a retired commander with the Chicago Police Department.

Tony Bertucca: Tony played professional football for the Chicago Bears and is a former Chicago Police officer.

Father Dan Brandt: Dan is an ordained priest of the Catholic Archdiocese of Chicago. Dan is the full-time director of the Chaplains' Unit for the Chicago Police Department.

Lenny Cacioppo: Len is a retired Chicago Police officer with over thirty years of service; he was an HBT Swat Sniper, Special Operations officer, and firearms technician.

Chris Cinnamon: Chris is an exercise physiologist, lawyer, author, wellness expert, and head instructor at Chicago Tai Chi.

Rosa Cortez: Rosa is a holistic health practitioner and the founder of Naperville Healing Center, LLC. She is a 10 Generation Mayan Healer and the founder of The International School of Healing & Yoga.

Denise M. Coyle, LMFT, CTS: Denise is a regional clinician for the Drug Enforcement Administration (DEA) in Seattle. She is a licensed marriage and family therapist.

Thayer Crouse: Thayer is the Director of Development and Outreach for Chateau Recovery in Midway, Utah.

Kimberly Lewis-Davis, DMin: Kim is a Chicago Police Department chaplain and police officer. She earned her doctorate of ministry degree from United Theological Seminary.

Sonja DePratt: Sonja is a licensed clinical social worker with twenty-five years of experience. She is certified in Internal Family Systems (IFS).

Jack A. Digliani PhD, EdD: Jack is a licensed psychologist and a former law enforcement officer. Dr. Digliani is the author of *Reflections of a Police Psychologist, Contemporary Issues in Police Psychology,* and the *Law Enforcement Peer Support Team Manual.*

Ed Epstein: Ed is a neurofeedback coach at the Advanced Neurodiagnostics Institute for Clinical Applied Neuroscience.

Phillip S. Epstein, MD: Phil is a University of Chicago Pritzker School of Medicine graduate, was a Fulbright scholar in neurochemistry and cofounded Midwest Neuropsychiatric Associates.

Luke Fairless, PsyD: Luke has a doctorate in clinical psychology from Adler University. He is on the Illinois Department of Corrections Staff Wellness Response Team.

Dr. Marla Friedman, PsyD, PC: Marla is a police psychologist and a national trainer. She is the current chairman of "Badge of Life™" and developed the health protocols for their "Building a Better Cop" program. She is the author of *Processing Trauma: Cognitive Behavioral Therapy*.

Tom Grutzius: Tom is a police sergeant in law enforcement.

Adrienne Gardner: Adrienne is a lieutenant in the Richmond Virginia Police Department and has a master of science degree in criminal justice from Virginia Commonwealth University.

Kurt Gawrisch: Kurt is a Chicago Police officer with a master's degree in clinical psychology from Concordia University. He holds certifications as a CIT Officer, CIT State Instructor and CIT Coordinator.

Joe Gentile: Joe is a retired Chicago Police officer with over thirty years of experience and was a hostage negotiator and CIT instructor.

Kevin Gilmartin, PhD: Kevin is a behavioral scientist specializing in law enforcement and public safety related issues. He is the author of the book *Emotional Survival for Law Enforcement: A Guide for Officers and Their Families*.

Nicholas Greco, MS, BCETS, CATSM, FAAETS: Nick has a master's degree in psychology, is a board-certified expert in traumatic stress, and is a fellow at the American Academy of Experts in Traumatic Stress.

Kevin W. Graham: Kevin is a well-respected Chicago Police officer and the past president of Fraternal Order of Police, Chicago Lodge 7.

Justin Gruby, DC, CKTP: Justin has his doctorate of chiropractic medicine. He is board-certified in integrative medicine.

Dan Herbert: Dan is a former police officer and Cook County prosecutor. Dan has over twenty years of experience with Dan Herbert Law Firm.

Carol Henderson: Carol is a clinical hypnotherapist and a certified EFT practitioner, and has been with New Day Hypnotherapy, LLC, in the Kansas City area. for almost twenty years.

Michael Hughes: Mike is a retired detective with the Chicago Police Department.

Stephen James, PhD: Stephen earned a doctorate in Criminal Justice & Criminology from Washington State University in 2015. He is a research specialist in sleep deprivation.

Olivia Johnson, DM: Olivia is the founder of the Blue Wall Institute and holds a doctorate degree in organizational leadership management.

Mike Jones: Mike is an ordained minister certified in critical incidents, stress management, and suicide.

Mike Kehoe: Mike is thirty-seven-year law enforcement professional and retired as police chief of Watertown, Connecticut. He was the police chief at the time of the Sandy Hooke Elementary school shootings.

Hyun Kim: Hyun is the owner of Naperville Mediation in Naperville, Illinois.

Gary Kujawa, MS, LPC, NCC: Gary is a Chicago Police officer with an MS in clinical mental health from National Louis University. Gary is a licensed professional counselor and a nationally certified counselor.

Michael Lappe: Mike has been in law enforcement for over thirty-four years and is an elected Board Trustee for the Policemen's Annuity and Benefit Fund of Chicago.

Bob Lindsey (aka Coach Bob): Bob is a forty-five-year police veteran and member of the International Law Enforcement Educators and Trainers Association.

Al Lopez: Al has been a Chicago Police officer since 1972, and he retired in 1999. He has been a Chaplain with the Chicago Police Department since 1982.

Beth Medina: Beth is the CEO of the Innocent Justice Foundation and the program director for SHIFT training. She holds a master's degree in marriage and family therapy.

John Marx: John is the executive director of the Law Enforcement Survival Institute (LESI) and author of the book *Armor Your Self™: How To Survive A Career In Law Enforcement*. He served twenty-three years in law enforcement.

Matthew May: Matt is a captain in the Wake Forest Police Department. in North Carolina. He has a bachelor of arts degree in Justice and Public Policy from North Carolina Wesleyan College.

Doug Monda: Doug is a retired Cocoa Beach (Florida) Police Department officer and speaker on police suicide and PTSD.

Ben Pearson, LCSW: Ben is the clinical director for Chateau Recovery in Midway, Utah.

Timothy F. Perry, Rev.: Tim is the creator of Nationwide Chaplains and 10-41 Incorporated.

Victoria Poklop: Vickie is the police counselor with the Des Plaines Police Department, and she received her master's degree in counseling from Indiana University.

Lisa Proctor: Lisa is the chief of police of the Kings Mountain Police Department in North Carolina.

Antonio F. Pugliese, DN: Antonio is a licensed acupuncturist and board-certified in Naprapathic Medicine. His practice is Driven Wellness in Franklin Park, Illinois.

Dara Rampersad, PhD, LPC, NCC: Dara is a first responder and forensic psychologist, and licensed counselor. He is certified in Crisis Intervention Teams (CIT) as a CIT Coordinator. He owns and operates BluePaz First Responder Services.

Laura Rufo: Laura is a Reiki master and teacher. She is enrolled at Midwest College of Oriental Medicine for acupuncture and she holds a BA from Colombia College.

Jeff Sachs: Jeff is a sergeant with the Chicago Police Department.

Christopher Scallon, MPsy: Chris is a retired sergeant with over twenty-four years in law enforcement with the Norfolk Police Department. He holds a master's degree in psychology and specializes in Critical Incident Stress Management. He is the founder of Survival Mindset Training and Consulting, director of Public Safety Support for Chateau Recovery, and is IACP Vicarious Fellow.

Jonathon Sheinberg, MD, FACC: Jon is a lieutenant on the Lakeway, Texas, Police Department, a fifteen-year United States Air Force veteran, and received his medical degree from Georgetown University in Washington DC.

Bruce A. Sokolove (Coach Sok): Coach retired with forty-three years in law enforcement He has a master of science in Police Administration/Public Safety and is the deputy director of Badge of Life.

Eric R. Ramirez-Thompson, PhD: Eric earned a doctorate in Criminology, Law, and Justice from the University of Illinois at Chicago in 2019, and is a criminal justice instructor at the College of DuPage.

Frank Scarpa: Frank is a lieutenant with the Richmond, Virginia Police Department.

Christopher Taliaferro: Chris is the 29th Ward Alderman on Chicago's City Council and chairman of the Council's Committee on Public Safety. Chris is also an attorney, a former Chicago Police officer, and a Marine.

John M. Violanti, PhD: John is an internationally known expert and researcher on police stress. He retired with twenty-three years in law enforcement as a New York State Trooper. He is a research professor of epidemiology and environmental health. John has written and edited seventeen books on police stress.

Duane Wolfe: Duane retired from his career as a Minnesota Peace Officer after more than twenty-five years of service. Duane has a Bachelor of Science degree in Criminal Justice from Bemidji State University and a master's degree in Education from Southwest State University.

Rabbi Moshe Wolfe: Moshe is a Chicago Police chaplain for over thirty-five years and a Chicago Fire department chaplain for over twenty-eight years. He graduated from the Rabbinical College in Cleveland, Ohio.

Doug Wyllie: Doug has written many articles ensuring the well-being of police officers, including an article in 2019 for *Police Magazine* titled, "3 Keys for Financial Wellness for Police Officers."

Ronald A. Rufo EdD

Working for the Chicago Police Department for twenty-two years was an honor and a privilege. I retired in 2015 from the 18th District. I spent most of my career as a crime prevention speaker in the Preventive Programs Unit. It was through good fortune that I received specialized training in suicide prevention and became a certified member of the Chicago Police Department Critical Incident Team.

The city of Chicago has a tuition reimbursement program, which I was fortunate enough to utilize. It was not easy going back to college at age forty-one, but I did it. What an exciting day when I received my bachelor of arts degree in criminal social justice and graduated with highest honors and earned the designation of Scholar of Lewis University in 2000. My mom and daughters were there that memorable day to celebrate with me.

I was inspired by watching the graduating master's students receiving their graduation hoods. I again enrolled in the post-graduate program at Lewis. Many of my fellow students were half of my age, but that made me work harder. I graduated in 2002 with my master of arts degree in organizational leadership. I was hoping to eventually make sergeant.

I soon learned that a cohort was forming to attend Argosy University for their doctoral program. I was one of twelve officers and supervisors accepted into this prestigious class. I was blessed to have a wonderful chairman and mentor, Dr. Paul Busceni, who guided me through everything that was required to attain my doctoral degree. There were times that I wanted to quit. I was frustrated and felt the uphill battle was too much. With the encouragement of my wife, Debbie, I defended my proposal and research with flying colors.

One of the proudest days of my life was the day in 2007 that I received my doctorate degree in organizational leadership from Argosy University. My dissertation topic was *An Investigation of Online Sexual Predation of Minors by Convicted Male Offenders*. I thought the world should know how devious sex offenders can be and decided to write my first book, *Sexual Predators Amongst Us*, which was published in December 2011 by CRC Press, part of the Taylor Francis group.

I met a truly remarkable professor when I was an instructor for the master's program at Kaplan University. Dr. Lauren Barrow and I decided to coauthor a book on criminal profiling. The name of our book is *Police and Profiling in the United States: Applying Theory to Criminal Investigations*, and it was published in 2012 by CRC Press.

I was involved in peer support early on in my law enforcement career. I was honored to become a peer support team leader a few years later. It was through peer support that I became interested in the subject of police suicide, and why so many officers were taking their lives. What was the problem? My third book, *Police Suicide: Is Police Culture Killing Our Officers?* was published by CRC Press in August 2015. I am wring this book on police wellness to give my fellow officers a resource to a better life on the job and in their retirement.

I have been busy in my retirement. I am delighted and privileged to be a keynote speaker with Badge of Life. This is a great organization that helps fellow officers in need. I have three beautiful daughters, Rita, Laura, and Cara, and a wonderful granddaughter named Alinah. I love them all with all of my heart. I am married to Debbie, who has always stood by me through thick and thin. I have a passion for antique cars, and I love my red 1959 Cadillac convertible.